In Praise of *The Bloom Book*

"*The Bloom Book* offers a vision of a new future and then helps to walk us there with flower essences as an intermediary. With equal parts evidence, faith, and personal experience, Heidi clearly lays out a path of personal healing connected to collective and planetary healing. This book was not what I expected; it's much more than a primer on flower essences and a glossary of how to use them. Heidi ambitiously and thoroughly spans the origins and histories of vibrational medicine and social justice theory, as well as herbalism, to make this a contemporary, relevant, progressive, and beautiful resource."

KIMBERLY ANN JOHNSON
author of *The Fourth Trimester*

"Heidi champions a voice for the flowers that is at once intelligent and intuitive, deeply heartfelt, and immensely insightful. Her knowing is authentically experience-based as she shares the journey of her own soul transformation as well as those of her clients. She also reaches widely into the network of practitioner research in flower essence therapy, distilling and synthesizing information into her own unique and credible approach. *The Bloom Book* is not a book you will read once and store on your shelf; rather it is a living source that you will return to again and again for inspiration and practical application."

PATRICIA KAMINSKI
founder of the Flower Essence Society, author of *Flowers That Heal* and *Flower Essence Repertory*

"Until I sat down with this book, I had not ever really considered what soul work is and how it could help others. Like many people, I've sometimes dismissively associated a lot of aspects of self-care and psychic healing. I was surprised to immediately connect with Heidi's ideas not to understand everything exactly (that would be the journey, right?), but to want to understand even more about myself and our world on psychic and cosmic levels. And yet that makes the end goal sound self-serving, which it is not. What Heidi presents is a story of how the world, and all of us along with it, got so out of whack. She is worried and passionate about inequity, imbalance, and the interplay of misogyny, racism, and privilege with the innermost aspects of individuality. Her writing is transportive but still accessible, even on the most mind-blowing of notions (quantum reality, vibrational medicine). Her learning, which she invites you to use as your own teaching, is deeply personal and duly engaging. And her book, best of all, is a work of hope."

CLAIRE HOWORTH
executive editor of *Vanity Fair*

"*The Bloom Book* offers a pathway to healing that could lead to our collective transformation. Heidi Smith makes flower essences accessible through clear and engaging prose that grounds what could be a very esoteric topic in relevant history and the urgency of now. This gorgeous book should be read and returned to again and again by anyone interested in evolving through this present moment to manifest a world that is more just, whole, and interconnected."

AIMEE MEREDITH COX, PHD
anthropologist at Yale University and author of *Shapeshifters*

"A wild ride. This book was written with a conscious mind. It is innovative and informative as well as enthralling and provocative."

PATRICK FRATELLONE, MD, RH (AHG)

"In these very turbulent times, Heidi's book is a clarion call for us to return to our essential nature through plant medicine and a realization of the wisdom of divine feminine energy. *The Bloom Book* is a wonderful offering to everyone who is working to bring their life back into balance. It guides us from ego to heart center—a vantage from which we can really show up for ourselves and for our fellow humans on this planet."

RAGHU MARKUS
executive director of the Love Serve Remember Foundation

"Heidi Smith has written a verbal and visual masterpiece. She writes from a perspective of guiding the reader toward the energetics within and around us and how to identify, accept, and positively affect them for ourselves and those we seek to heal. For laypersons and practitioners alike, Heidi digs into that which we cannot see but most certainly can feel, sense, and imagine in a way that teaches and guides. This book offers a depth of understanding and resulting confidence that will leave you wanting to add flower remedies to both your personal healing kit and that of your patients."

DR. PENELOPE MCDONNELL, ND

"Flowers are gentle yet powerfully restorative—containing the highest healing vibrations of all plants, having a subtle, profound effect on our health and well-being. Heidi Smith's beautifully written *The Bloom Book* is an invaluable guide for those of us who wish to explore the process of self-discovery through the vibrational healing of flower essences in a clear and accessible way."

JULIE ELLIOTT
creator and founder of In Fiore

"Heidi Smith has created an invaluable resource for personal and spiritual growth in *The Bloom Book*. She demystifies the intricate world of flower essences—steeped in ancient wisdom stretching from all corners of the earth and various healing modalities, yet accessible and approachable. It reads as a warm, open invitation back to a world in balance with the plant kingdom."

ALISON CARROLL
founder of Wonder Valley

"*The Bloom Book* is a deep and profound offering of healing in collaboration with Mother Earth. With a truly holistic, honest, in-depth, and beautiful layout, this book will act as an ongoing ally to readers as they grow through the wisdom, practices, and rituals offered. The historical and social context is refreshing given our current political, environmental, and social climates. I highly recommend this book for anyone who is ready to enter into new levels of consciousness and heal in relationship with themselves, their communities, and the Earth."

VANESSA CHAKOUR
herbalist

"This is the book on flower essences that I've been waiting for! Heidi Smith emphasizes the importance of setting intention with plant work and letting your intuitive force guide you in the process. These words, alongside those charming illustrations, have resonated with me more so than any other book on flower essences that I have come across so far."

SPENCRE L.R. MCGOWAN
certified herbalist, author of *Blotto Botany*, and creator of Gingertooth & Twine

"Heidi focuses on flower essences as a way to work through ingrained traumatic familial and societal imprints that lead to destructive belief systems. These belief systems can become psycho-spiritual conflicts embedded in the physical body as expressions of unresolved wounds. With her practical and deeply thoughtful book, Heidi draws us back to the power of plants and flowers to transform us—to be subtle partners in healing not only our own personal wounds, but the larger collective and societal ones as well."

JON KEYES, LPC, NCC
herbalist

"Heidi Smith's transformative practice-oriented book marries a deeply holistic and self-actualized approach to personal healing and growth with an incredibly thoughtful understanding of the power plant medicine offers us. Her intuitive and inspiring methodology is sure to help us all dive more fully into the pursuit of cultivating collective well-being through more immersive explorations of how we integrate flower essences into our own practices. The intention and expression of this book is as engrossing as it is enriching, a must-have for anyone seeking to deepen their understanding of the healing power right outside our doorsteps."

GRETCHEN JONES
strategic business advisor and Neuro-Linguistic Programming practitioner

"A provocative and thoughtful book that will inspire the next generation of herbalists and individuals looking to bring the art and magic of flower essences into their everyday lives. It's a wonderful offering for those looking to live with a deeper connection to the intricate energies of the universe, a love poem to this mysterious life in all its glory."

JOVIAL KING
founder of Urban Moonshine

The Bloom Book

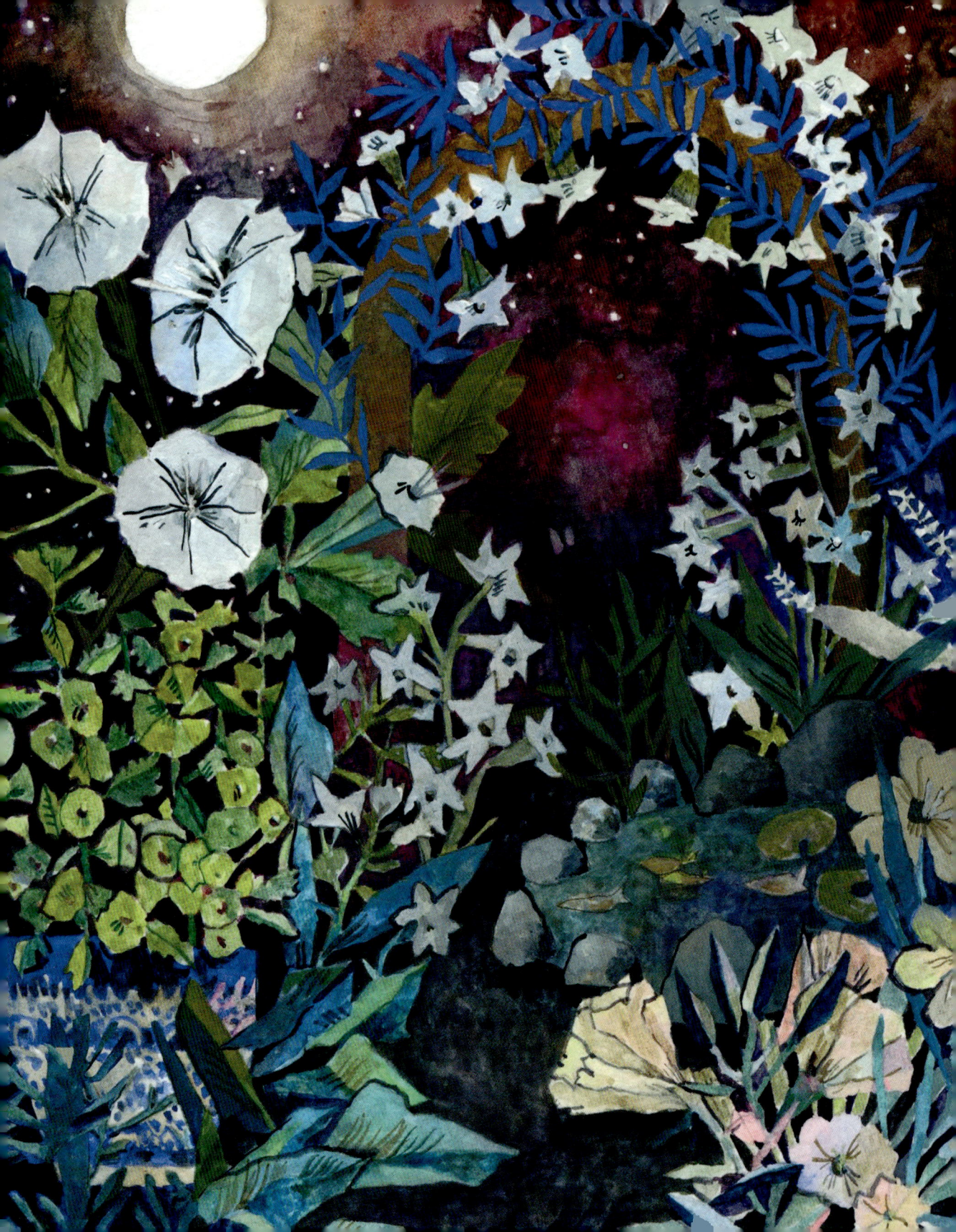

The Bloom Book

A FLOWER ESSENCE GUIDE TO COSMIC BALANCE

HEIDI SMITH

ILLUSTRATIONS BY CHELSEA GRANGER

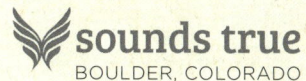
BOULDER, COLORADO

Sounds True
Boulder, CO 80306

© 2020 Heidi Smith
Foreword © 2020 Jane Bell

Sounds True is a trademark of Sounds True, Inc.
All rights reserved. No part of this book may be used or reproduced in any manner without written permission from the author and publisher.

This book is not intended as a substitute for the medical recommendations of physicians, mental health professionals, or other health-care providers. Rather, it is intended to offer information to help the reader cooperate with physicians, mental health professionals, and health-care providers in a mutual quest for optimal well-being. We advise readers to carefully review and understand the ideas presented and to seek the advice of a qualified professional before attempting to use them.

Published 2020

Cover and book design by Jess Morphew
Illustrations and cover image © 2020 Chelsea Granger

"Alchemists Collecting Dew" image on page 101 reprinted with permission by Alamy Stock Photo.

Printed in South Korea

Library of Congress Cataloging-in-Publication Data

Names: Smith, Heidi (Therapist), author. | Granger, Chelsea, illustrator.
Title: The bloom book : a flower essence guide to cosmic balance / by Heidi
   Smith ; illustrated by Chelsea Granger.
Description: Boulder, CO : Sounds True, 2020. | Includes bibliographical
   references and index.
Identifiers: LCCN 2019022805 (print) | LCCN 2019022806 (ebook) | ISBN
   9781683643807 (hardcover) | ISBN 9781683643814 (ebook)
Subjects: LCSH: Flowers--Therapeutic use.
Classification: LCC RX615.F55 S65 2020 (print) | LCC RX615.F55 (ebook) |
   DDC 615.8/515--dc23
LC record available at https://lccn.loc.gov/2019022805
LC ebook record available at https://lccn.loc.gov/2019022806

10 9 8 7 6 5 4 3 2 1

*This book is dedicated to my brother, Stuart,
who set me on my path.*

Contents

Foreword | ix
Jane Bell of
Presence of Heart

Preface | xiii

CHAPTER ONE | 1

Introduction and My Journey

How to Use This Book

An Intentional Invitation

CHAPTER TWO | 11

Coming into Cosmic Balance

From Moon Times to Sun Times

Divine Feminine Consciousness

Out of Cosmic Balance

Return to Cosmic Balance

Choosing Conscious Beliefs

Focusing

The Role of Relaxation

Radical Self-Care

Being of Service

Healing for Ourselves,
the Collective, and the Planet

CHAPTER THREE | 51

The Blooms

What Are Flower Essences?

How Flower Essences Work

Herbal Medicine

How Nature Heals

Vibrational Medicine

Cultural Appropriation and Colonization Within Western Herbalism and Flower Essence Therapy

Selection and Application: The Language of Plants

Formulation: How to Make Your Own Medicine

Women Healers Throughout History

The Foundations of Flower Essence Therapy

Color Theory and Rainbow Consciousness

The Flower of Life

CHAPTER FOUR | 125

Flower Rituals for Healing and Transformation

The History of Flowers in Healing Traditions

Safety, Protection, and Psychic Hygiene

Working with Intention

Abundance and Privilege

The Moon, Medicine, and Ritual

Dream Work

Heart Medicine Rituals

Tend and Befriend: Circling Together

Conclusion: Flower of Life Activation

Acknowledgments | 182

Appendix | 183

Notes | 186

Glossary | 196

Resources | 204

Index | 209

About the Author | 213

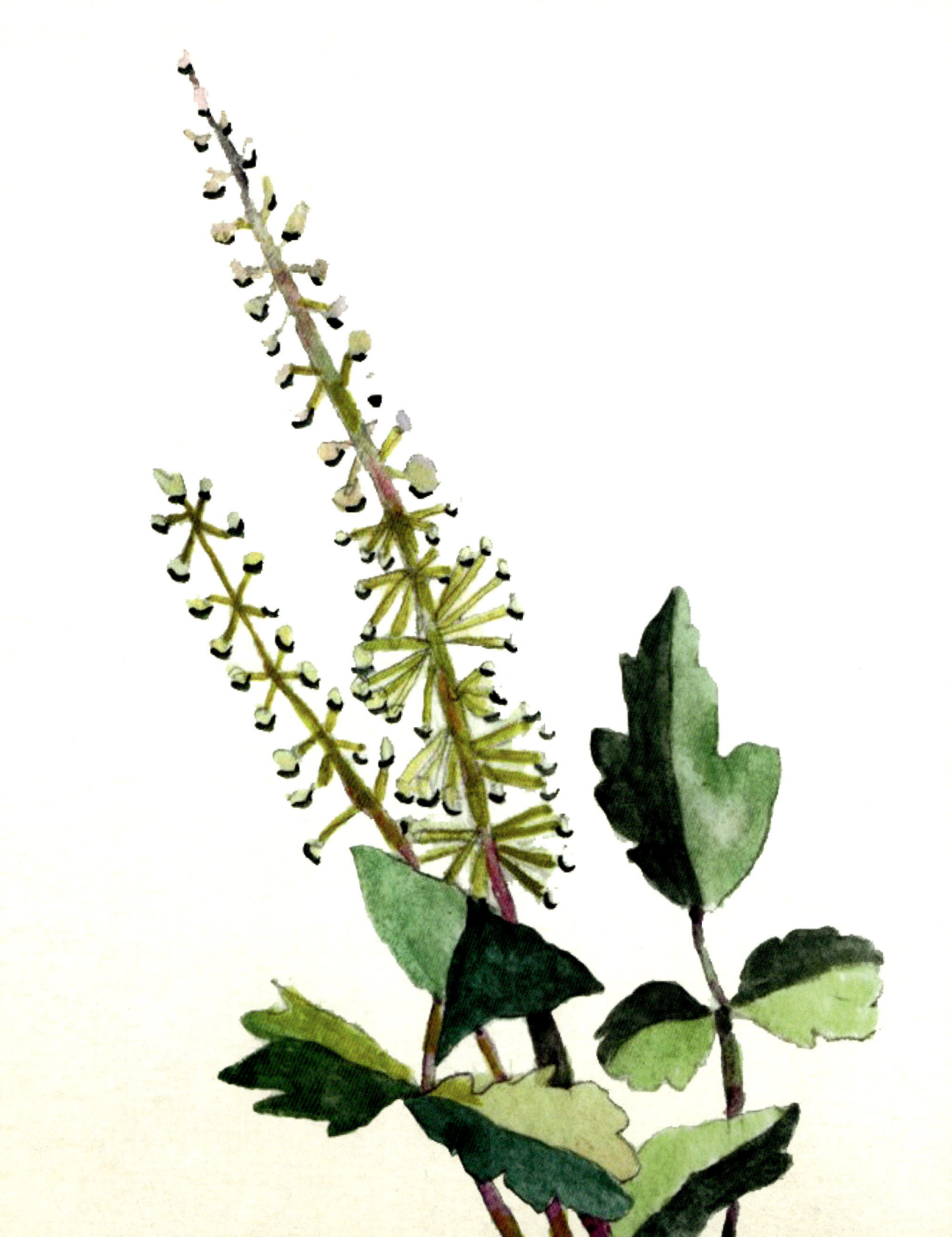

Foreword

AFTER FORTY YEARS OF meditation and spiritual practice, working with others in ceremonies, mystical journeys, and private sessions, I met Heidi Smith. The introduction came from David Groode, a mutual friend and intuitive, who had suggested that Heidi and I work together. We had an initial meeting at my healing center in San Francisco just before she moved to New York City. Then, for seven years, we met every week for one hour on the telephone. I had never had a student more focused, dedicated, and deeply interested in spiritual evolution than she was. Her commitment to awakening the divine feminine within her grew out of her discovery of her own self-worth and value. As she healed herself, her desire to share her own understanding with others became imperative.

In this text, Heidi covers a broad history, offers tools for personal development, and imparts her passion for the unseen realms of the plant kingdom. She incorporates her understanding of the ancient mystical teachings with the shamanic wisdom of the indigenous peoples. Her fresh perspective to awakening the divine feminine and plant consciousness is what makes this an important book.

Heidi offers us an opportunity to examine ourselves. She gives us a historical context for the exile of the feminine in our culture as well as an intuitive understanding of the importance of integrating our temporal selves and our transcendent ones, our feminine aspects and our masculine ones, our mystical nature and our linear minds. We have learned since birth about splitting ourselves, often judging and blaming what we can't understand or appreciate. We have a difficult time admitting our mistakes or failings, often blaming them on others for fear of shame or humiliation. The patriarchy has made vulnerability a sign of weakness rather than wisdom, so people work hard at hiding their true selves rather than being honest about their imperfections.

Our society values money over authenticity, fame over service, adoration over self-love. With *The Bloom Book*, Heidi has given us a way to intersectionally find and honor all the feminine aspects that we have learned to dissociate, denigrate, and diminish. Out of these chapters we rise up and meet ourselves fully, consciously, and with a toolbox that allows us to be fully integrated humans capable of traversing all realms of consciousness. This book is a personal guide full of understandings that brought Heidi to her own calling: helping people awaken to their own path by working with the unseen teachers of the plant kingdom. Her offerings here empower us to follow our own inner call, our own heart's desires—and in so doing we can find a way to heal not only ourselves but the Earth as well. Nothing is more compelling than learning from the devas and spirits of the plant kingdom, who shine a light on our understanding. The answers we seek lie in all of nature and the Earth we inhabit. The indigenous people of this Earth have always known this; they have honored the animal and plant kingdom as holy spirits. Our insistence on striving to conquer and own our dense material world has destroyed the very place we need for our survival.

The message in *The Bloom Book* empowers us. We recognize that everything is not as it seems. Heidi's own personal guides from the hidden realms taught her about vibrational medicine, healing, and the power of plants. After many years of hard work, she began to trust the voice within and followed the guidance that emanated from there. She also sought out mentors and teachings to enhance the information that came from her own direct experience. Heidi has the capacity to challenge and question her assumptions. She seeks not just to reinforce her own answers but also to challenge them. What she presents here is written with authority and humility.

It is a privilege for me to introduce this book to you. I am so proud of this woman, who, with immense courage, has stepped through many challenges to write with great clarity and passion. I am inspired by her and have great faith that because of her, and others like her, the ancient wisdom will come to light—not in the cloistered world, but for all of us to understand and incorporate into our daily lives.

Jane Bell
Presence of Heart

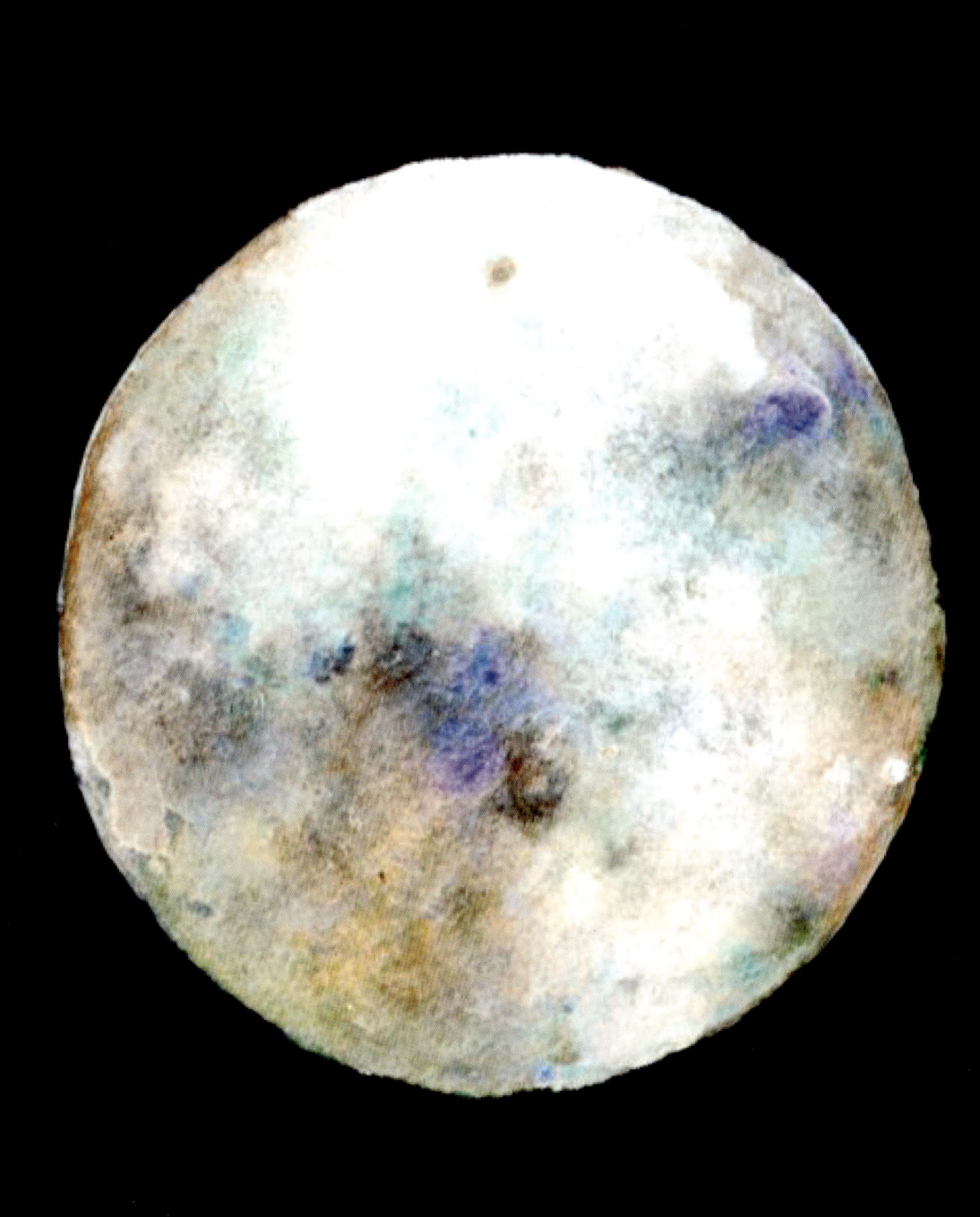

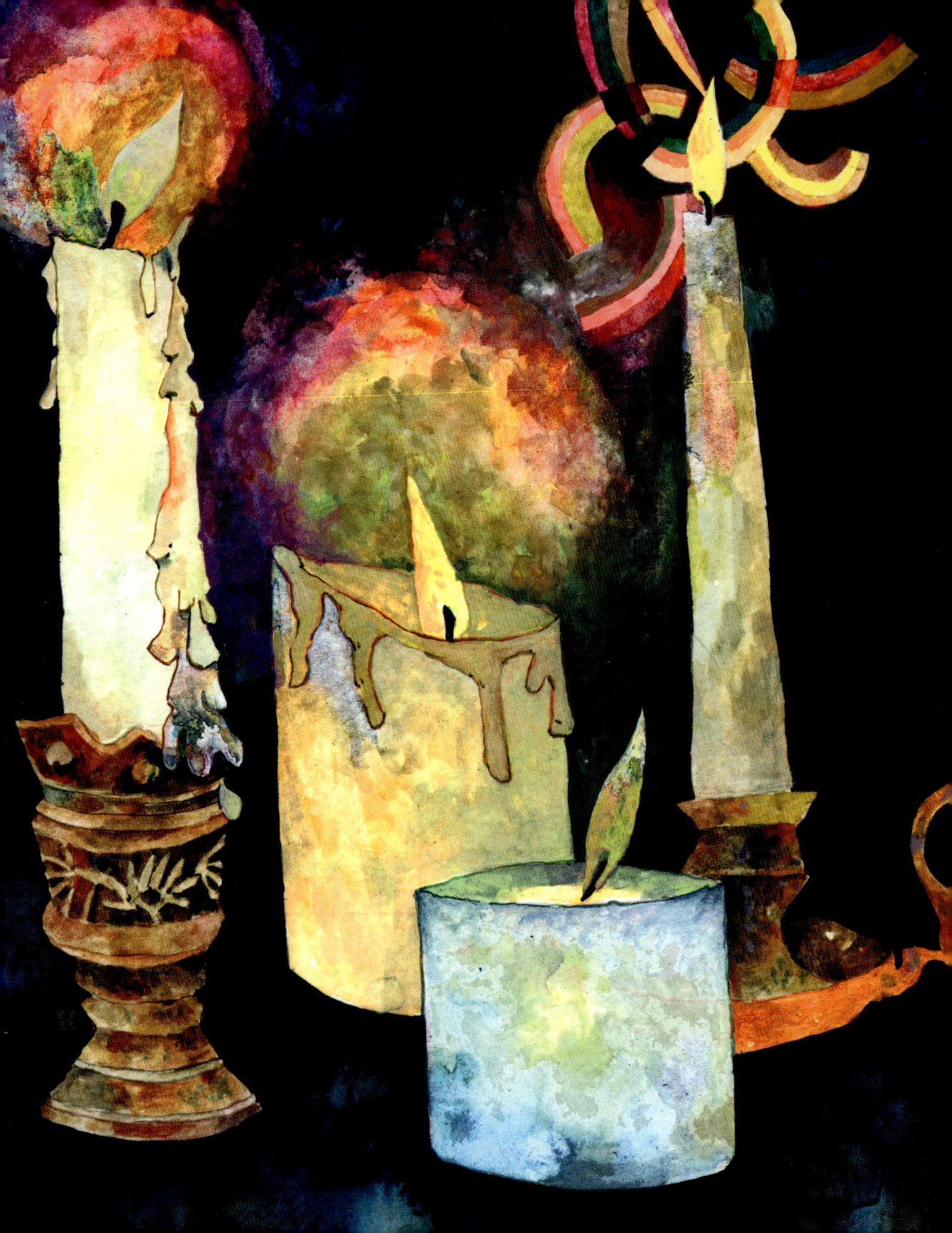

Preface

WHEN I FIRST STARTED this text, in the summer of 2016, I was filled with great hope that positive global change was imminent. Much has happened in the last few years for me, the collective, and the Earth. I am even more heartened in knowing that individual and collective change is not just possible, it is indeed occurring at a quickening pace. *The Bloom Book* exists as a guide for those who feel called toward the flowers to heal, transform, and evolve. Since starting this project, I am even more clear in my guidance from the plants: they are here to help us wake up and heal ourselves, each other, and our sacred Gaia. The ascension of this planet is happening; the process is accelerating even as you read this book.

Let's start here: what we believe affects how we feel and function. In order for me to discuss how flower essences work and why we need them, it's necessary for me to elucidate just how ingrained a lot of harmful beliefs have taken root in our psyches. So I will discuss how duality and the patriarchy affect how we feel and how we heal. Another way to understand the awakening process is a return to alignment, and it happens not in a vacuum but on a quantum level—each part affects the whole and vice versa. We are each a microcosm of the macrocosm, and this thankfully is coming into clearer view with the increasing awareness of intersectionality and social justice.

Poet and activist Emma Lazarus wrote, "Until we are all free, we are none of us free."[1] Our liberation is connected collectively, and with freedom comes responsibility: for ourselves, for all sentient beings, and for the Earth. The Earth is asking us via the plant kingdom to take responsibility with increasing urgency. Many of us weep for the Earth and her inhabitants because of escalating instability. The flowers continue to show me that this process, though horrifying and heartbreaking, is part of a natural cycle. We do have the opportunity to be in flow with this task, making heart-based decisions (as opposed to dualistic, fear-based ones) that make a positive impact.

Thinking beyond limiting constructs and questioning what we think we know grants us access to subtler and subtler levels of healing—something for which the flower essences are exceptionally attuned. I am not asking for your permission to speak my truth within these pages. But I am asking, humbly, that you receive my offering with an open heart and mind.

For now, allow me to introduce where the doorway to the flowers first opened for me.

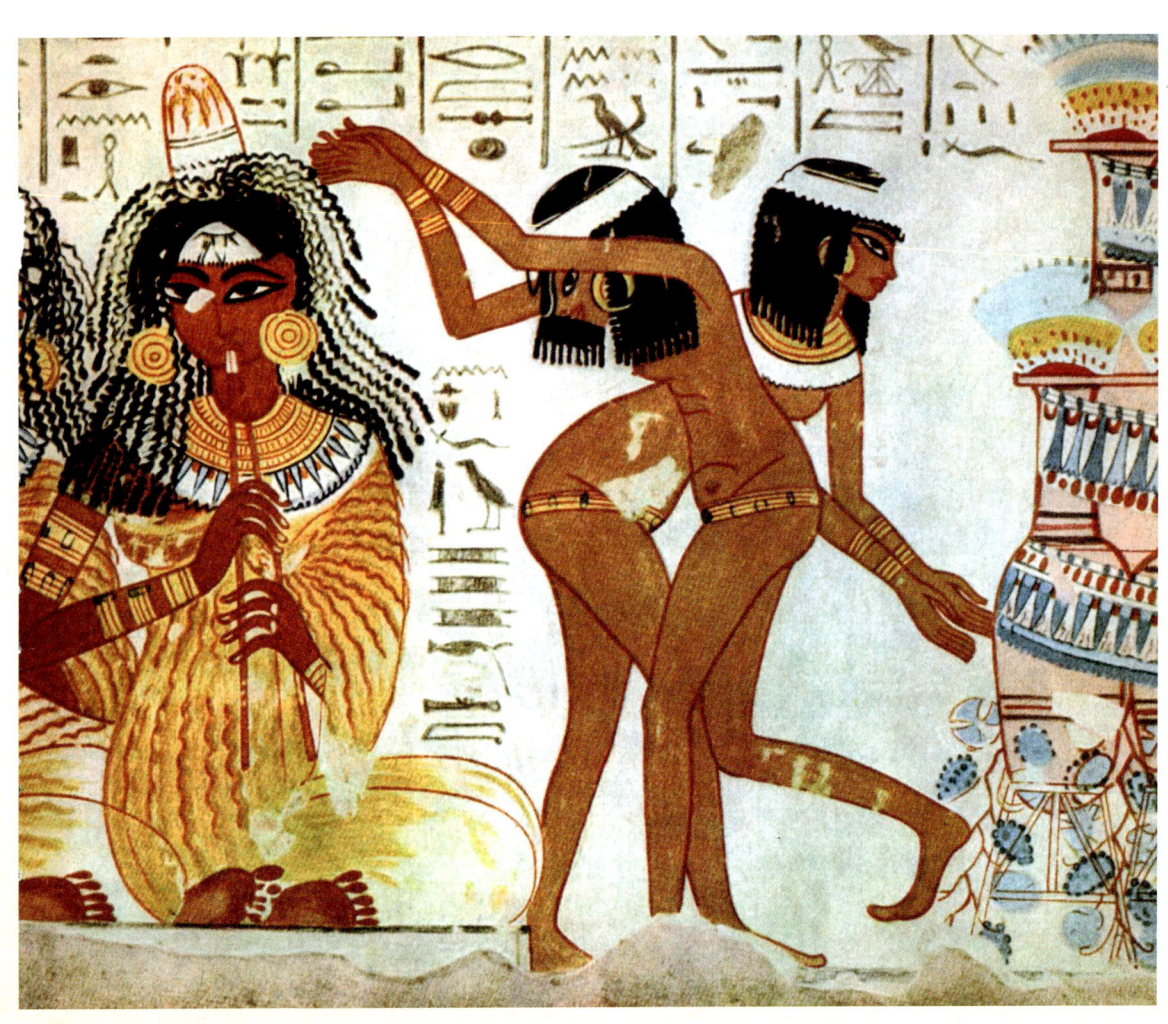

CHAPTER ONE

Introduction and My Journey

If you have come here to help me, you are wasting your time. But if you have come because your liberation is bound up with mine, then let us work together.

Lilla Watson

LIKE MANY SEEKERS, I was motivated by pain and existential confusion to find deeper answers for my suffering. When my younger brother committed suicide in 2007, David Groode, a trusted friend and intuitive, introduced me to mimulus, a Bach flower remedy that is meant to help alleviate fear. I didn't know what it was or how it worked, but once I started taking those drops three times per day, I knew they were helping me move forward despite my intensifying anxiety. Since then, I keep several flower remedies in my medicine kit. David also introduced me to Presence of Heart founder and spiritual teacher Jane Bell. Jane would become my mentor and guide for the next seven years.

When I met Jane in 2007, I felt I had found the candle that would illuminate my path forward. With her guidance, we traversed the terrain of my wounding and underlying belief systems. We plumbed the depths of my psyche and found the shadows of the universal consciousness—patterns and programs ingrained in all beings that could be healed and cleared with intention, commitment to the process, and love. My transformational growth was exponential when I traveled with Jane to Egypt—a pilgrimage to the ancient holy sites that still resonate with the divine wisdom frequency of the mystery schools. Those sacred temples and the people I met there changed my heart consciousness forever.

In graduate school, studying psychology in the Western mode, I struggled to resolve what I knew about the nature of reality from my mystical studies and what was presented by the medical/academic model. I felt there was so much more to life and healing than merely talking about our physical issues. It also became evident early on that, while I was studying social justice and healing, a lot of the academic structures perpetuated—rather than challenged—gender and racial bias.

The bridge I had been waiting for—to connect what I knew on a soul level, and what I was called here to do, with academic theories I learned from Carl Jung to Carl Rogers—came in the form of a book given to me by my future husband. It was Gurudas's *Flower Essences and Vibrational Healing*. Gurudas authored several of the earliest books on vibrational medicine with the help of channeler Kevin Ryerson. For me, at that time in my life, the book, although extremely "out there," spoke to the vibrational nature of all life.

Vibrational medicine uses specialized forms of energy to positively affect those energetic systems that may be out of balance due to disease states. Flower essences work with higher levels of consciousness, the subtle bodies, the chakras, as well as the physical and biomolecular form.[1] When I refer to flower essences as "subtle," I mean that the way they work is energetic and may or may not produce physical effects. The process of working with flower essences can be as gentle as drinking chamomile tea or it can gong you as hard as a psychedelic experience. Flower essences connected me: with healing, with others, with the evolution of the planet, and what I now know as the collective consciousness. They also reinforced my vision of ascension—we come here to be in our hearts and evolve. Later, I realized that, while returning to school proved to be an enriching and invaluable experience, in truth I had gone there asking the patriarchy for permission that it would not and could not grant: to allow me to be an integrative therapist who uses flower essences. The answers weren't there, and the doors were closed. So I sat by myself and waited.

The next two years were the hardest of my life. (My astrology during this time was off-the-charts horrible!) On the surface I was functioning, but on the inside I was falling apart. Despite years of training and study, I had reached what I would later understand to be a dark night of the soul. I felt like the worst version of myself. As brutal as that time was, I now know I had signed up for that experience. I recognize that I was in a position of privilege to be having that experience and could rely on family, friends, and my partner to help me through that time.

Through all of this, with presence and acceptance, I continued to stare at the moon, wondering what she had in store for me next. And I carried my flower remedies with me in my medicine bag, trusting I wasn't going through it alone. And, sure enough, the tides began to shift and the planets changed course.

In 2014, I was fortunate enough to find another teacher, Claudia Keel, an herbalist and flower essence practitioner. My apprenticeship with Claudia accelerated my learning dramatically, bringing me out of a self-led, self-taught period of exploration and into a time of fellowship, mentorship, and application.

Suddenly my dream of working with the flowers was very real. So, on the new moon of July 2014, with the support of my teachers on Earth, Jane and Claudia, and my guides, I launched my private practice, which I named Moon & Bloom. Within months, I had a roster of beautiful, brave, and highly conscious clients who humbled me with their teachings even as they learned from me—and I finally felt at one with my dharma.

So here we are.

This book is the realization of the assignment I was given by the Universe: to bring people to the flowers and to serve as a guide for greater alignment and heart consciousness. The purpose of this book is to bridge cosmic insights from the divine feminine* and the flowers in an accessible language for people who are not afraid to excavate in order to heal deep below the surface. It is for those of us who are committed to creating positive shifts within the problematic status quo, and who understand that change begins with challenging our own inherent duality. It is not a book on this-for-that flower remedies to merely suppress uncomfortable symptoms. With this book, you can access insight from other realms in a grounded way to navigate within the physical world.

It is likely our Earth will continue to become a more challenging place to exist, so we will all have to be increasingly better-resourced to survive and thrive, and to teach our children to do the same. Every lifetime affords us the opportunity to gain new experiences and polish a facet of our multidimensional beings. Everyone gets a piece of a puzzle, and it is our contribution to evolutionary transformation. This book is my piece of that puzzle I offer to you.

In choosing to incarnate as humans right here, right now, we agreed to participate in the split between masculine and feminine consciousness: the separation,

---

* Language note: This text centers on all women and divine feminine energy. I use masculine and feminine to denote energetic characteristics, not to reinforce the gender binary or heteronormativity. I do discuss the feminine/masculine binary throughout this book as this dynamic is part of creation and nature; nature is differentiated, it only becomes negative when it's within an oppressive system. Energy may be masculine, feminine, both, or neither. I do discuss the moon as being a symbol of the sacred feminine, as that is my experience of it. That said, the moon has no gender, and everyone's experience of it is subjective.

black and white, right and wrong, human and divine, mind and body. This duality underscores much of the conflict within ourselves as well as the chaos and corruption in our world today. It's a crazy time to be on the planet! It comes with great responsibility and great opportunity. Now, perhaps more than ever, we have the ability to create our reality on a grand scale. We all have a role to play in the cosmic unfolding. We are all called to reconnect with our divine natures. This is the way forward—we must learn to exist in our hearts, connect to our inner light, and heal our relationships to ourselves and the Earth. Flower essences can help.

While many ancient cultures exhibited greater harmony with nature, our modern civilization has overvalued masculine qualities (achievement, aggression, competition, objectivity, and so on), creating a toxic, fear-based society. To develop integrated consciousness is to progress from separated, physical, egoic masculine consciousness into more balanced, integrated, heart-and-soul awareness—all qualities typically associated with the divine feminine.

As I will explain, we come from divine consciousness, but have been in the Dark Ages, so to speak, and are transitioning back into a lighter time—a time of heart-and-soul consciousness.* Finding a balance between the divine feminine and the divine masculine energies and achieving equilibrium between these two paradigms is essential for our individual and collective evolution as well as for the health of our planet. Taking it a step further, we must open our minds to thinking beyond this construct, beyond the level of masculine and feminine altogether. By making space for all parts of ourselves and the human experience—the seen as well as the invisible realms (of which flower essences are a part)—we gain access to the infinite, and all the possibilities therein.

Much of what I offer in this text is nothing new. It is information that has been protected and transmitted through various lineages of the divine feminine throughout history. The divine feminine invites us to remember the language passed down by the goddesses, priestesses, deities, *neteru*, devas, bodhisattvas, *curanderas*, witches, and wise-women healers. These transmissions communicate with us via a vocabulary many already use, including alternative health practitioners, doulas, massage therapists,

---

* Some esoterics and traditions believe the Earth goes through 12,000-year cycles, called yugas, oscillating between masculine and feminine energy. Some individuals and groups who subscribe to the belief of the 24,000-/12,000-year Earth cycle are: Yogananda Paramahansa, Rudolf Steiner, Edgar Cayce, ancient Egyptians, several ancient branches of Hinduism and Tibetan Buddhism, Maya, Inca, and Hopi.

teachers, activists, and healers of all kinds—people with a commitment to justice and higher consciousness in environmental, economic, political, and social realms.

All forms of alternative medicine are becoming increasingly popular, and flower essence therapy contains special gifts to share with us around how consciousness heals. More and more people are beginning to question the Western/allopathic medical model in favor of more integrative and natural approaches. Science continues to "prove" axioms that ancient systems have long held about healing, such as how being in right relationship with the natural world improves our health.[2]

Flowers represent a branch of plant medicine that is specifically concerned with our consciousness and evolution. Chronologically, flowers developed after the mineral kingdom and came into form later on in the plant kingdom—as such, their energetic signature, or healing ability, is finer. Flowers hold a special affinity for the finer subtle physiology of the self: the subtle bodies, chakras, and our conscious development. Flower essences, or remedies, offer a vastly different healing experience than taking a pill to alleviate a physical symptom. Since I conceptualize all life vibrationally, I write from this level, which I hope will resonate with many psychically and emotionally sensitive beings.

Flowers exist within a multidimensional rainbow, as do humans. Every flower holds a unique consciousness, and to connect with it is to connect with the unique healing available within that frequency. Flower essences deal with our attachments to certain disease states and life situations, allowing us to gain awareness about how and why certain things occur within and around us. They offer a different perspective on our healing journeys so that we can step back and make healthier, more integrated decisions. Since they are actually more of a process than a medicine, flower essences pair well with any complementary, mindful, or spiritual practice you may have, and are best understood through your subjective experience.

All plant medicine links us with the natural world. This happens in a dramatic way via the heart, which connects directly with nature and the cosmos. Flower essences play a special role in expanding heart consciousness: with their help, we can more powerfully give and receive love, exist in a state of unconditional love and forgiveness, and work in the flow of co-creation with all life. When we work with flower essences, we engage a process of self-discovery, of validating ourselves and our experiences. We link very powerful nonphysical considerations to our physical health, such as our ancestral history, our dreams, supernatural phenomena, and intuitions—things that are generally not part of a standard medical intake, but nevertheless offer highly valuable insight into who we are and how we experience the world.

I spend a good amount of time in this book offering background information on vibrational medicine and the belief systems we've been indoctrinated with concerning healing, because what we believe has a huge impact on our health and well-being. We have to revise our understanding of healing and wellness. Our attachment to duality plays a big role in this. The tension between masculine and feminine consciousness extends into the Western medical model. In Western medicine, mechanical (masculine) and holistic (feminine) philosophies are presented in opposition. The truth, however, is that there is a place for empiricism as well as qualitative and phenomenological analysis in all medicine, including flower essence therapy. Both are valid; both sides are necessary for seeing flowers' potential.

Plant medicine has always been the people's medicine, and flower essences create unique opportunities for issues surrounding accessibility, as essences are extremely safe and can be made rather inexpensively. The shift toward holism—complementary and alternative medicine (CAM) and integrative medicine—and the proliferation of herbal interventions within our health-care system are proof that we are making progress. In light of this, there are a number of dynamic ways we can promote flower essences to be even more accessible and inclusive for people. Even flower essence therapy itself is a modality historically dominated by white men, but increasingly it is being pushed forward by women-identified, LGBTQ, and POC healers.

The injury Western medicine forces upon marginalized groups spills into alternative medicine as well. Herbalism and flower essence therapy are included in this reckoning. Increasingly, the alternative healing community is processing its own biases. Much of alternative medicine was developed in the service of the dominant culture, or the patriarchy. Therefore, it hasn't been a healing space for many groups, including but not limited to women, people of color, LGBTQ, people with disabilities, economically oppressed people, neurodiverse people, and (in the United States) non-native English speakers. In the words of Cara Page, a founding member of Kindred Southern Healing Justice Collective, healing justice "identifies how we can holistically respond to and intervene on generational trauma and violence, and to bring collective practices that can impact and transform the consequences of oppression on our bodies, hearts, and minds."[3]

One of the main themes of this book involves balancing duality, which means challenging the perpetuation of oppressive systems. Unless we are actively engaged in dismantling racism, sexism, homophobia, transphobia, xenophobia, and ableism, we are merely reinforcing the power structures we are claiming to challenge. As models of healing justice are emerging, many organizations and community collectives are generating their own missions and value statements from which to work. Meanwhile, practitioners like me have to ask themselves, "How is my work a function of my privilege? Where are my blind spots? Does my practice truly support inclusivity, diversity, and accessibility?"

The working definitions of healing and trauma are also evolving. Within a healing justice framework, one can see how, by understanding trauma merely as "an emotional response to a terrible event," we are ignoring a more inclusive interpretation that includes the cumulative and historical trauma of colonization. In the last decade, science has "validated" that trauma is intergenerational and historical. Likewise, many traditions include community in what constitutes emotional and spiritual healing, whereas Western models of mental health are focused exclusively on the individual self.

In this way, it is an exciting time for the community of herbalists and flower essence practitioners. Modalities that are so helpful in bringing people into balance are themselves coming into greater balance. A sign of hope within an era of great hope. Even if the clinical data for flower essences and other CAM cannot compete with the pharmaceutical industry that dominates the clinical trials and studies, the ancient wisdom explored in this book supports that the power of the plants is coming through in dynamic new ways. This text exists, in part, to provide more context around the validity and potency of the flowers. The spectrum of human emotional experience is here for our development and delight. The flowers are here to support all the colors of the collective rainbow!

How to Use This Book

I created this book to be a source of information and light. The flowers exist, in part, to assist us in evolving—both individually and collectively. This text contains aspects of healing that I explore in both my personal and clinical practice; I believe the flowers to be powerful helpers for rebalancing the collective. Much of what I present here is highly subjective, and it's up to you, the reader, to find the truths that align with you. While I offer possible interpretations and solutions, you get to decide what information, ideas, and practices are for your highest good.

I will also offer flower essence recommendations, which are completely optional, but you are certainly invited to follow along experientially. You don't need to go out and purchase all the flower essences I suggest to benefit from the text. You may choose to use the suggestions for reference, or for deeper study, and come back to them later.

An Intentional Invitation

Working intentionally is a theme that will come up throughout this book. Energy follows intention, and working with intention is no small thing. Naming the state you want to bring about in your life is a first step toward real change. Intentionality has become one of the most powerful pieces of my transformation and is essential to all parts of my spiritual practice. When you begin working with intention, you will see the energetic seeds you sow mature into very real plants.

As you begin using this book, I invite you to take some time to set a few intentions of your own. In my experience, working intentionally with reading materials ripens the possible fruit they can bear. What would you like to get out of your time with this book? Perhaps you would like more practical information about flower essences, or maybe you have a particular issue you're struggling with and would like to use this book as a way to address it. It's possible you're not sure why you picked up this book, and maybe your intention is to allow your curiosity to guide you into greater consciousness.

If you feel called, you could say a prayer, affirmation, or mantra, such as, "I will use this book for raising consciousness to honor my soul's highest good." Any and all intentions are welcome!

Every chapter contains several creative exercises to engage your right brain (feminine, intuitive, subconscious hemisphere), inspire, and encourage deeper study.

The artwork was created collaboratively with artist Chelsea Granger. This book contains contributions by several other healers who work with flower essences in their practices. It is with great joy that this text includes the wisdom of my fellow light workers!

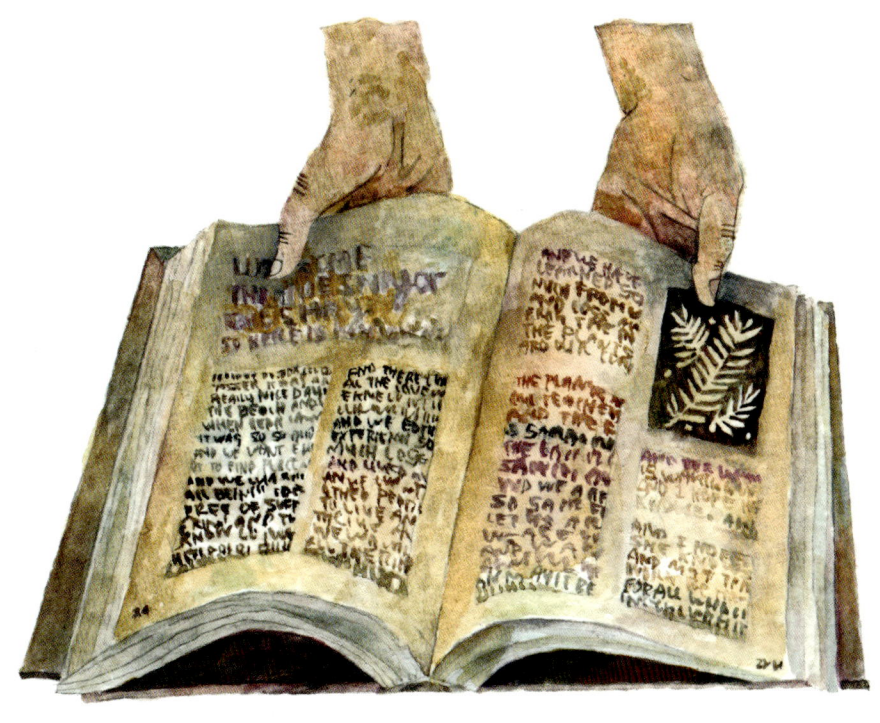

EXERCISE | Setting Intention

What would you like to get out of the time you spend with this book? What are you curious about? What do you hope to learn, to feel, to understand? How does that look? How does that feel in your body and in the field around you?

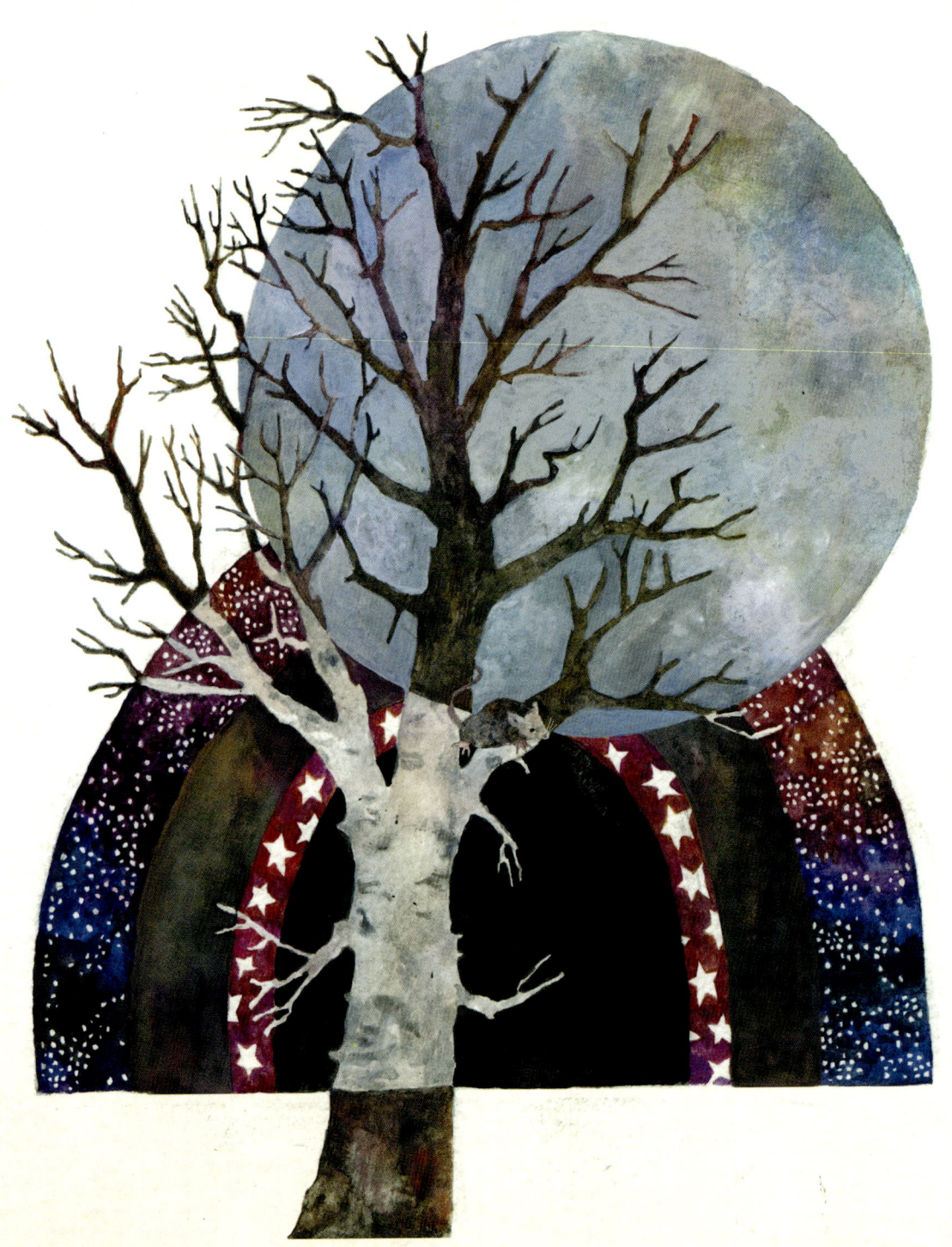

CHAPTER TWO

Coming into Cosmic Balance

WE HAVE ENTERED A TIME of massive transition from a masculine paradigm to a feminine era. We are moving from separation to unification, and it is a time of both extreme volatility and miraculous potential. That the patriarchy is an oppressive force is not a new concept. But now, there is a cosmic rebalancing underway, and all the disowned and denigrated aspects of the feminine, within ourselves and the Earth, are rising. I'm interested in the genesis of this phenomenon because I think it sheds light on *what* we were connected to before this, *who* we were before this, and *where* we get to make different choices in light of knowing our true roots and our true history. What's in our DNA and consciousness that remembers the truth? A way back into our hearts? Into alignment? As I will explain, the flowers are here to help us in this rebalancing mission since much of the disease states we experience are a result of this separation from divinity, from nature, and from our true selves.

This chapter explores some of the main ways we've fallen out of equilibrium and some ways that lead back into balance. Nature is our biggest teacher for living in harmony with our environment. Our beings also contain the harmonic codes for cosmic balance, which the flowers assist us in activating by way of shifting our consciousness. This process affects us all, and the balancing of the toxic masculine is very much an energetic healing crisis that has been underway for millennia and is the root cause for many of our healing journeys.

From Moon Times to Sun Times

In addition to working with plant medicine, I want to look at the effect patriarchal domination has on our health, individually and collectively. The healing work many of us have embarked on is not relegated to our lifetimes only; we are healing many generations of ingrained toxicity and disease. Flower essences really shine as awakeners of awareness; and being aware of how our civilization fell asleep shows us where we need to shine the most light in order to heal. In my work I continue to find that we are all negatively impacted by the patriarchal, or toxic masculine, paradigm, and the resulting denigration of the feminine—regardless of race, class, gender/nongender-conforming, ability level, cultural background, or sexual orientation. I've created a couple of charts in this chapter to break down the differences in these paradigms, and to show some of the aspects of what a balanced or exalted state could look like.

I utilize the metaphor of the moon to symbolize the feminine, and the sun to symbolize the masculine. The moon has always been a prominent figure in folklore. It exists in a constant state of cyclical transformation, as do we. We can learn much of what the moon meant to the ancients based on their creation myths. Regardless of geographic location around the ancient world, the symbol of the moon represented similar ideas: death and rebirth, creation, and power.

The Hebrew calendar is based on lunation, and many ancient rites were organized around the cycles of the moon. In ancient Egypt, the moon was "thought to be the carrier of the souls of the dead over waters to the sun."[1] As Jules Cashford shares in *The Moon: Myth and Image*, without electricity and nothing to dull the night sky, the moon must have been spectacular in the ancestral environment. The moon's beams were potent medicine for conception, divination, and healing.[2] Myriad ancient tales from around the world hold that at some point a split occurred between the sun (which represents the masculine) and the moon (which represents the feminine).

While the vast majority of our modern world's religions contain a tremendous amount of misogyny, there are a few wonderful exceptions. Several examples of more matriarchal-focused prehistoric civilizations existed in parts of Asia and Africa. In Nigeria, the Yoruba tradition features a rich matriarchal mythology, and its creation story attributes all life originating from an androgynous deity, Nana Bùrúkú.[3] My teacher, Jane, introduced me to the ancient Egyptian mysteries, which exemplified a matriarchal-patriarchal balanced civilization—a perfectly harmonious state of being known as Ma'at. It's hard to overstate how exciting it was for me to learn about an ancient civilization that existed outside the toxic masculine paradigm!

The Earth has gone through many iterations. From the myths, we can see the progression from unity consciousness (sun and moon are in union, humanity is divine) to split consciousness (moon is opposing sun, humanity is egoic). According to some, there were two major shifts away from perfect cosmic balance. The first split in consciousness can be characterized by the shift from unity into duality and separation. Theoretically, it occurred between Lemurian and Atlantean times, and this duality manifested as a separation between body and mind, humanity and the divine, man and woman. The second shift into greater separation, after the fall of Atlantis, occurred during the epoch of the Holy Roman Empire. This time the natural world was divided into physical (valid) and subtle (invalid). With this development, the divine feminine and nature consciousness assumed a subordinate position to the masculine. We see a proliferation of dominator cultures/religions, colonization, and the moon retreating behind the sun. Here are some of the differences between moon times and sun times.

Moon Times	Sun Times
Matrilineal focus	Patriarchal focus
Exalted feminine	Denigrated feminine
Women embody their bodies	Women disembodied, shamed; men have ownership
Integration of subtle and physical bodies	Overidentification with physical and mental bodies
Integration of rational and nonlinear	Overidentification with linear and rational mind
Awareness of the collective unconscious	Conscious = real, unconscious = invalid/bad
Connection to dream world, spirit world	Emphasis on physical world
Night	Day (night becomes bad)
Darkness, shadow	Light (darkness and shadow become bad)
The Great Mother	Father God

Moon Times	Sun Times
Priestess	Priest
Maiden-Mother-Crone	Virgin-Whore split
Earth in balance with cosmos	Humans dominate top of the pyramid life
Respect for all beings	Emergence of "isms": racism, ableism, heterosexism, and so forth
Creation	Possession
Collective responsibility	Individual rights
Elements in harmony, balanced yin and yang	Overabundance of earth and fire elements, excess yang
Abundance	Scarcity/lack
"I am because we are," Zulu proverb known as Ubuntu	"I think therefore I am," René Descartes

Throughout history there have been numerous ethnic and cultural groups that were matrilinearly organized. This was the case for many Native American tribes such as the Cherokee, Hopi, Iroquois, and Navajo. Over time, matriarchal-balanced societies became more patriarchal. With the rise of capitalism, women and nature became entities to be conquered and dominated.[4] The collective moved into a time of the sun, an era of the toxic masculine. The moon was now in opposition to the sun, representing the crazy, the darkness, the hysterical, the taboo, the void. It became associated with the occult, magic, and witches, all of which were deemed evil. "The *Malleus Maleficarum*, the great and hideous Catholic treatise against witchcraft, insists that demonic powers are 'deeply affected by certain phases of the Moon.'"[5] The moon was vilified through its association with menstruation, which was considered unclean.

Yet pockets of protected moon wisdom remained, by virtue of the keepers of the mysteries and indigenous groups, a few of whom maintained their sovereignty despite the larger societal shifts toward patriarchal domination.

Our history is a biased chronicle written, in large part, for and by white men. The burning of the library in Alexandria in ancient Egypt has been a constant reminder

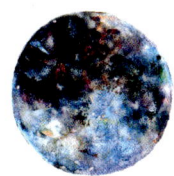

throughout history that physical remnants of the truth can be destroyed, and the past becomes revisionist instead of reality.

Our history books offer a perfect example of such revisionism. They make the founding of America sound predestined and noble. However, when we apply a more objective historical analysis, the American story takes on a very dark tone. In reality, this country was founded by enslaving millions of people and exterminating millions more.* A capitalist economy like ours incentivizes a dominator culture to take power over vulnerable populations through violence and appropriation. The devastating effects of colonial oppression cannot be overstated. We are all holders of this violence and trauma both ancestrally and energetically, as is evidenced by neuroscience and epigenetics.[6]

And yet, while our beings have been inundated with the toxic masculine for millennia, we also contain the light codes of the divine feminine and unity consciousness. The plants hold so much wisdom for us to tap into for this process of unification and waking up.

While you do not need to embrace a different interpretation of our beginnings to use flower essences, it's a worthwhile exercise to consider because it is very likely that flower medicine evolved simultaneously in our collective development, in accordance with a different history than the version we have been taught.

Whenever I work with a client, I always assess their case from this historic contextual level because what we believe plays a huge role in how we feel and how we heal. For instance, I recently began working with a woman who, despite all her extensive healing work and professional success, had persistent symptoms of powerlessness and depression. Over time, she was able to identify that in her family and culture of origin, she was not seen as special and accomplished because women in her family

---

* All white people enjoy a great deal of privilege as a result of colonization, slavery, as well as current institutional racism, whether they are aware of it or not. Being aware of one's privilege is one powerful way to dismantle patriarchy. This can be very painful yet rewarding and, ultimately, necessary work. Additional information on this topic can be found in the Resources section.

were not allowed to be proficient in anything. Her success equaled literal abandonment by her father. This program (a set of ingrained, harmful beliefs) was not merely informed by her family but by our culture as well. It was useful for her to address and see how this occurs collectively and is embedded into our ancestry, in order for her to observe this phenomenon objectively, as opposed to believing it was her fault and her responsibility to "fix." In this case, cerato essence—one of the first essences I often give people to assist in trusting themselves—helped her to discern her truth within this pattern and free herself from the cycle of disempowerment.

Divine Feminine Consciousness

The ancient tales and goddesses remind us that we are descendants of an infinitely wise matriarchy. Highly sophisticated cultures in antiquity—the energetic lineages of which are still alive today in many non-Western modalities and traditions—are examples of this level of awareness. The divine feminine is nothing new; in fact, it arises out of reverence and remembrance of the ancients' wisdom and mythology.

What exactly is consciousness? Philosophers, writers, and scientists have attempted to define consciousness, and most descriptions tend to be too mechanistic. Modern science would like us to believe that consciousness occurs only in the brain and only in humans. Here's my take: consciousness is a state of awareness that can occur in multiple levels and dimensions simultaneously and is not limited by time or space. Everything with a vibrational signature possesses consciousness. This includes but is not limited to: the elements, the oceans, the cosmos, places, memories, disease, feeling states, plants, stones, and animals. Though consciousness is more defined than *un*consciousness, they are both part of the great mystery.

Feminism and divine feminine consciousness are similar constructs under which to observe what is occurring to society as a result of patriarchy. I prefer to work from the definition of feminism posited by psychologist, Dr. Carol Gilligan. "Feminism is one of the great liberation movements in human history. It is the movement to free democracy from patriarchy. In that sense, it's a movement to free everyone from the gender binary and the hierarchy of patriarchy in the interest of women and men, in the interest of love. It is a way of dealing with human conflicts other than through the use of force and the imposition of hierarchy."[7] And if feminism exists to liberate

A FEW MOON GODDESSES
FROM AROUND THE ANCIENT WORLD

In Northern Europe: The British Isles are famous for their faerie lore and are thought of as one of the bastions of Atlantis. The faerie folk do most of their work outdoors under the auspices of the moonlight. They especially love to sing and dance under a full moon. The Celtic moon goddess was Rhiannon.

In ancient Greece and Rome: Selene, Artemis, and Aphrodite; Luna, Diana, and Venus. Also, the Virgin Mary, Black Madonna, and Black Virgin.

In the Middle East: Hathor/Isis and Lilith.

In Asia: White Tara, Tibetan, Quan Yin.

In India: In Hindu, Shiva was the witness and vibration, represented by the moon.

In Babylonia and Assyria: Ishtar or Mari.

In Africa: Oshun and Oya.

In Sumeria: Inanna was also the goddess of sex and war.

In the Americas: The Mayans regarded the moon goddess Ixchel as a companion and evil aspect of the sun, with a crown of serpents. They regarded the moon as a symbol of idleness and promiscuity. The Aztecs saw the moon as a daughter of the rain god Tlaloc.

---

everyone, then we must make it intersectional*, centering on those who have historically been marginalized, and taking into consideration race, class, sexual orientation, age, disability, and gender. .

I feel a kinship with Gilligan's interpretation of feminism because it feels close to the way I define divine feminine consciousness: a paradigm of awareness that applies

---

* Intersectional feminism is a term created by Kimberlé Williams Crenshaw in 1989.

ancient, sacred feminine wisdom for the purpose of healing and transformation. Divine feminine consciousness seeks to serve our ascension by the following:

- supporting a balance of the divine feminine and the divine masculine energies
- understanding the equilibrium between these two paradigms and holding space for all that is
- communicating with us via a language many already use, that of alternative health practitioners, doulas, teachers, activists, healers of all kinds, and people with a commitment to justice and higher consciousness across all institutions and systems (environmentally, economically, politically, and socially)
- connecting us with the wisdom of the ancients and applying previous teachings toward current and future evolution
- celebrating diversity and the higher qualities that connect us all
- cultivating our relationship to those qualities of the moon we've forgotten, especially the gifts of our intuition, creativity, receptivity, and our spiritual selves
- strengthening our relationship to nature
- allowing us to exist within our hearts
- understanding the true meaning of abundance

Divine feminine consciousness does not seek to blame the masculine or reinforce heteronormativity; it seeks to bring the masculine and feminine into balance and support the liberation of all beings. I am also not suggesting that the future is female or that we need to return to a matriarchy—this would merely be a binary and reactionary swing of the pendulum.

Regardless of gender or gender nonconforming status, we have all internalized the toxic masculine and the denigration of the feminine. Unworthiness is an especially Western malady that is a result of this imbalance, and it manifests within so many of us emotionally, physically, and spiritually. Balancing and transcending this polarity is a pathway toward unconditional love.

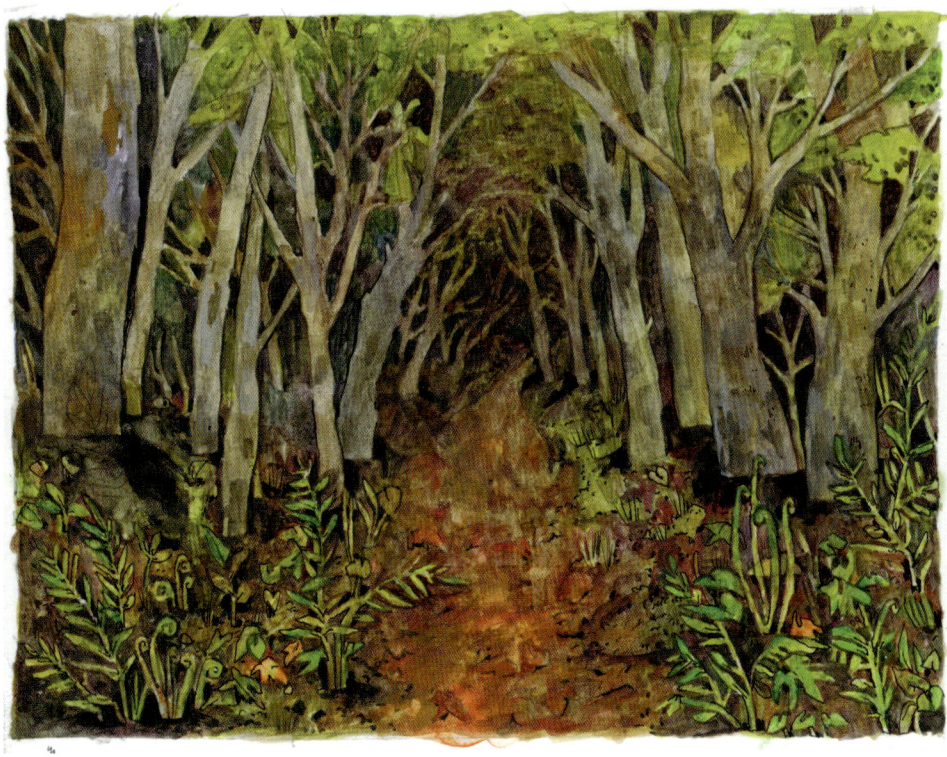

Out of Cosmic Balance

As we fell out of cosmic balance, we entered a time of separation, known as the Kali Yuga in Hinduism. Beyond the dualities, we are all unified: people, animal kingdom, mineral kingdom, and of course, the plant kingdom and the potentials of all the unknowns in our Universe.[8] Quantum reality is about conceptualizing life at the subatomic level. We must acknowledge the interconnectedness of all life.

Plant medicine has the power to bring us into balance with ourselves, with each other, and with our Earth. The ideas of balance and cosmic order are significant pieces of the mythology and creation stories of many ancient cultures. Ma'at was the ancient Egyptian goddess born from Ra, the sun god. She represented divine order; her symbol is a straight ostrich feather. Ma'at held the frequency of "as above, so below" and connected man with the divine through harmony. Most healing traditions hold balance as the key to optimal health. What manifests in our bodies often stems from what's going on "below"—in our thoughts, feelings, and emotions. The flowers can help us unify our bodies and our hearts. Likewise *tantra* is the unification of masculine and feminine energy within the *shushumna* (central channel of the body) to achieve inner peace.

I think most of us can agree that the dominant culture has evolved into a place of tremendous chaos. This imbalance and instability are crises of consciousness that are underscored by duality. Duality is the paradigm of awareness wherein everything is polarized as positive or negative, and conscious or unconscious. It is a binary system that reinforces male/female, right/wrong, black/white, self/other, yes/no, either/or, and so forth. There are endless dualities at the level of form, which is the current dominant state of being on Earth. Duality is a given condition of 3-D human life in many ways, but it is also necessary for us to think beyond this level. Quantum reality is the paradigm of awareness wherein everything is held in a unified field. Flower essences are subtle medicine that expand our awareness and bring us back into greater equilibrium.

Thinking dualistically is very harmful as it applies to race, gender, and sexual orientation. The white/nonwhite way of separating people is very problematic and reinforces the dominant white hierarchy, lumping all nonwhite people as "other." As it pertains to gender, reinforcing the binary system reinforces patriarchal masculinity. Those who identify as heterosexual and cisgender reinforce dominance, while all those who identify as LGBTQ, nonbinary, or nongender conforming are again separated into the "other" category. This otherness reinforces the good/bad paradigm and keeps us all limited from connecting to ourselves, each other, and all life with heart-and-soul consciousness.

The fact that the gender binary is breaking down and that intersectionality is now part of our vernacular is very encouraging. It means the collective is ready to question oppressive systems and think more quantum! We've been living in such an overtly masculine world for so long, but we are now entering into a more energetically feminine and gender-fluid time, and as this is happening, the illusion of existing only at this level is also emerging. As the masculine shows us the distinct parts, the feminine elucidates both the parts and the whole. The next stage, then, is thinking beyond, making way for infinite possibilities.

Duality and Nonduality

Nonduality/nondualism and duality/dualism are concepts that originate in Buddhist, Hindu, Taoist, many indigenous and shamanic teachings, and various esoteric and mystical texts. *Nonduality* means simply "oneness." Duality is a state of separation and can also be understood as a polarity, a tension of opposites, and binary consciousness.

Some Characteristics of Nonduality or Nondualism	Some Characteristics of Duality or Dualism
Oneness of all nature	Separation from nature
Dichotomies of self and other are understood as illusion; the ideas of holism, the microcosm and macrocosm, and unity consciousness	Separation from self and others
Past, present, and future all collapse into present time	Past or future time
Parts of the self are understood as interconnected and part of the whole (e.g., systems, subtle bodies, chakras, memories, emotions)	All parts of the self are separate; all beings operate as machines
Both physical and subtle anatomy are real and valid	Gross, physical anatomy is real; subtle, energetic anatomy is not real; physical symptoms are valid; emotional or spiritual symptoms are not valid (because they cannot be measured)
Conceptualization at the level of both/and	Conceptualization at the level of either/or
Masculine and feminine, intersex/queer/bisexual/nonbinary	Masculine or feminine; man or woman; cisgender or LGBTQ
Inclusivity	Exclusivity
Quantum understanding of reality	Reductionist, mechanical understanding of reality; Newtonian science

SYMBOLS OF
INTEGRATION

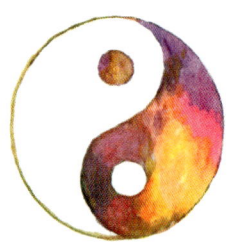

YIN-YANG

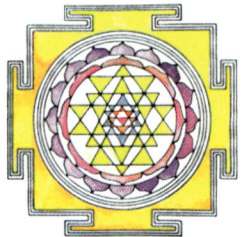

SHREE YANTRA

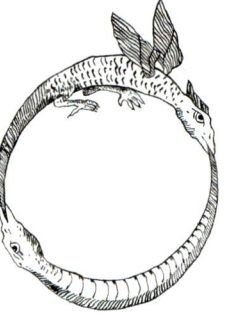

OROBOUROS

ANKH

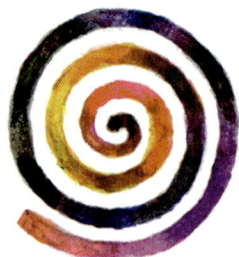

SPIRAL

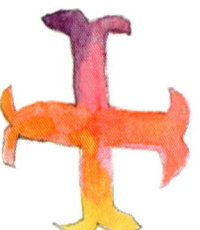

CROSS

The Power of Healing Duality

It is imperative for us to be aware of where duality lives within us. There is no separation between inner change and outer change. This is literally the way you become the change you want to see in the world; it's a quantum law. Gone unchecked, polarities either become unconsciously internalized or projected, creating negative quantum effects. Projection can happen at the physical and psychic level, and has very deleterious effects on our health and the health of our planet. Projection is essentially a way of avoiding accountability. It is the opposite of an integrated, balanced state. Polarities highlight the potential for balance and unity.

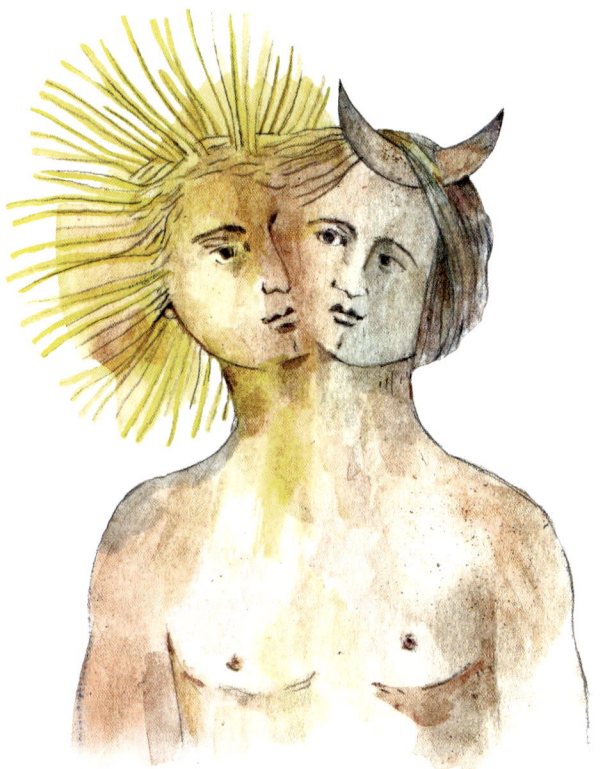

SUN AND MOON INTEGRATION

On a personal level, dualities inhibit our ability to recognize our whole multidimensional selves. Dual thinking keeps us perpetually locked in a cycle of positive or negative instead of being in balance. We are good or bad, worthy or worthless, beautiful or ugly, happy or sad. Or we are one-dimensional: beautiful but unintelligent, smart but ugly, successful but shrewish. Recognizing our internal dualities helps us to name all our parts and keeps us accountable. For example, think of a part of yourself you dislike. Can you name a positive aspect in addition to this part? Can you see yourself in terms of both/and instead of either/or?

Within the scientific and medical communities, we are in the midst of a sea change of redefining what is healing and why. Flower essences are both physical and vibrational agents of change. Both traditional empiricism and an expanded conceptualization of reality are needed to fully grasp their potency. In the last century, the proposition of the pilot wave model has revealed that the distinct nature between wave and particle does not exist at the subatomic level at all; instead light and matter exist as both particles and waves *simultaneously*.[9] The wave-particle theory is significant because, as science breaks down matter to the smallest possible measurable constituent—to the subatomic level—what lies beyond is the finding of the nondual nature of light and matter. With this breakthrough, science must reconcile that light and matter exist as both two distinct forms of energy at the same time, and may not exist separately at all. It is not either/or, it is both/and.

Lower Vibratory States

Much of our internalized duality manifests as problematic: thoughts, emotions, beliefs, and physical symptomology.* Lower vibratory states can be understood as difficult or uncomfortable emotional states or feelings. They can be situational, such as grief over the loss of a pet, or chronic, such as major depression. They are the resultant experience of trauma. Energetically, all emotional states exist on a spectrum and emit a frequency, a vibrational signature, just like plants. The frequency of feeling states can be

---

* I struggled with what to name this section because I really don't like to reinforce any emotions as negative. It perpetuates a good/bad binary, and it's not helpful to label some states as positive and others as negative. I also feel it's important to mention here that my work as a helper is not to reinforce an attachment (duality in disguise!), to merely feeling good, or to exist exclusively in higher vibratory states. My work is to help the self come back into balance through integration and engaging the heart. Healing on this level is soul work, and it is how we bring about true transformation and liberation. That said, coming into alignment does create more opportunity for higher vibratory states, such as love, joy, compassion, and gratitude. I've studied psychology and healing from both traditional and alternative orientations, and my understanding of this topic is very much a blend of the scientific and the spiritual.

MARIPOSA LILY

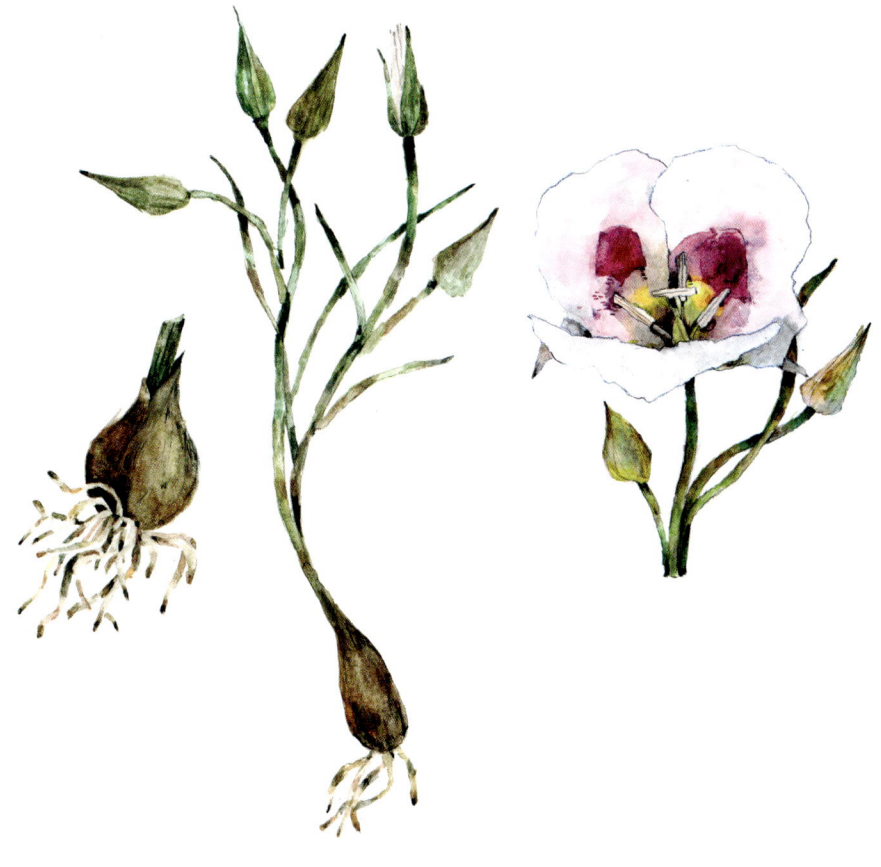

scientifically measured.[10] The lower end of the spectrum is characterized by fear; the higher end of the spectrum is characterized by love. Energetically, lower states can be felt as a contraction, whereas higher states can be felt as expansion. Most emotions generally fall under either fear or love; for example, if you hold intense anger for someone because they left you, underneath the anger is a fear of being abandoned, which is the root of the emotion. The following list illustrates the range of the spectrum, with "unconditional love" at the highest end of the spectrum, and "shame" at the lowest.

	Higher Frequencies
Unconditional Love	
Peace	
Joy	
Compassion	
Acceptance	
Neutrality	
Indifference	

Love ↑

Fear ↓

	Lower Frequencies
Stuckness	
Apathy	
Anger	
Desire	
Jealousy	
Sadness	
Loss and grief	
Hatred	
Guilt	
Shame	

In chapter four, we will explore low vibratory states in greater detail when we look at shadow work. I also include my top essences for lower vibratory states, which can be helpful to you as you navigate this terrain.

Trauma

According to Bessel van der Kolk, author of *The Body Keeps the Score*, "Trauma is an experience of helplessness and terror." It's an experience that affects how you perceive danger and results from "being in a state where you feel that nothing you can do can stop what's happening to you."[11] Our definitions of trauma are changing and becoming more inclusive. Indigenous Trauma Theory expands the concept to account for the lack of cultural context around colonization and the devastating impacts of ethnostress, soul wounds, and historical and cumulative trauma on indigenous people.[12] PTSD is probably the most familiar term for the emotional and physical symptoms that occur as a result of severe trauma such as war and rape. Vicarious traumatization describes the abuse sustained by working in a hostile environment, such as under a supervisor who is sexually inappropriate. Complex PTSD is a newer definition that includes five features: "emotional flashbacks, toxic shame, self-abandonment, a vicious inner critic, and social anxiety."[13] Adverse childhood experiences (or ACEs) are stressful or traumatic events that resulted from physical, emotional, sexual, or verbal abuse.*[14] It was previously assumed that sexual and physical abuse were most harmful to a child; however, as models of trauma evolve, we are learning that verbal and emotional abuse can be just as, if not more, deleterious to adult health. Personality disorders in particular are on the rise, and the prevalence of children with one or more mentally ill caregivers is likely higher than is documented.[15] Internalized duality is the trauma response, which manifests in many ways, and is almost always associated with lower vibratory states.

Energetically, trauma is imprinted somatically in our physical body and emotionally and psychically in our subtle bodies. It is not possible to heal trauma from just a logical, verbal orientation when our programs and stories become embedded. That is why mind-body-spirit integration techniques like the strategies mentioned in this text are so vital. Dr. Edward Bach, the founder of modern flower essences as we know them, was a bacteriologist and homeopath who, during his medical training in a hospital, observed that the "personality of the individual was of even more importance than the body in the treatment of his disease".[16] It was after his work with soldiers during World War I that he conceived of the first twelve flower remedies as a safe and natural alternative to address the shock and trauma of war.[17] He observed the correlation between personality and the incidence of certain illnesses and emotional symptoms. He also

---

* There is strong correlation between ACEs and mental and physical health.

discovered that, like homeopathic remedies, flower essences could resonate with particular states to affect healing change. We'll go into greater detail about Dr. Bach and how flower essences work in the next chapter.

Most of the time, trauma manifests as some sort of health challenge. Health challenges—emotional or physical—show up in the system because they want our attention; they want to show us where we can be in greater balance.* Many flower essence producers offer guides and texts to easily connect with the remedies for certain feeling states and life situations. These texts are provided in the Appendix.

Of the emotions on the challenging end of the spectrum, most people struggle with anxiety, depression, or both, either at some point in their lives or more chronically. Anxiety disorders are the most common mental illness in the US and worldwide, affecting approximately 18.1 and 8 percent of the population, respectively. Depression is the leading cause of disability worldwide.[18] One in six adults in the US regularly takes a psychiatric drug.[19] Clearly, the pervading scientific approach to mental illness needs to be reexamined. Being spiritual beings in a human body means feeling emotions—all of them. For those of us on healing journeys and who help others on theirs, I find it helpful to remember several points:

- Lower vibratory states are part of being human; there are no "bad" feelings. This includes very difficult states such as psychosis and suicidality.** Previously, the emotional body (the moon, the feminine) was seen as separate from the body and deemed negative. Naming and reintegrating challenging feelings is part of becoming whole, resolving inner duality, and coming more fully into one's power.

- As above so below, as within so without. If we live according to this precept, we know that whatever is occurring emotionally within us is the reality we create around us. For instance, if you hold much judgment for others, you will feel judged.

---

* Physical symptomology is always accompanied by some kind of emotional disturbance. Therefore, whenever you address a physical state of disease, you must always take into account the emotional body.

** Sometimes we feel suicidal. I take suicidality very seriously. Confronting inner annihilation is a doorway some of us must walk through, and it doesn't necessarily mean you are suffering from mental illness. If you feel unsafe, and if your suicidality is severe and persistent, it is always a good idea to seek support from a professional.

- All lower vibratory states are connected to beliefs and our inner child. These beliefs and feelings are ingrained and habitual. It is monumentally helpful to work with a practitioner to heal the relationship with your inner child, as this is the origin of most emotional imprinting.

- Nerve cells that fire together, wire together.* We all have emotional baselines. The more you feel a certain emotion, the more you create a natural baseline for that feeling state. The more healing work and therapeutic practices you utilize to bring yourself into balance, the more you have an opportunity to raise your frequency and create a healthier emotional baseline.

- While we all possess the ability to heal ourselves, we all need teachers and guides. This is especially true if you are dealing with seriously incapacitating emotions and addictions. Can you think of some people you can reach out to? Who's in your support team?

Above all, lower vibratory states and trauma are teachers. They are doorways into greater alignment. Can we be curious about them instead of fearing and labeling our negative emotions? They can also be mysterious and elusive. Sometimes, the process of alignment leads us to surrender. Surrender is an act of balancing inner duality because we consciously choose to detach from both the positive and negative polarity of our suffering. I discuss this later in this chapter, in the section titled "Relaxing into Presence and Acceptance."

While in the throes of my own serious depression, I eventually reached a place of deep surrender—letting go of the need to feel better, the need to know why I was still suffering, the need to control my journey. This process took many months, and eventually something did shift. Flower essences played a huge role in this shift by helping change my relationship to my pain, understand the stories and beliefs that were keeping me stuck, and calming very difficult symptoms. While I don't presume to understand all the mysteries of suffering and am not here to "fix" people, I have been given the opportunity to steward many clients through this process and believe that

---

* A fascinating development in addiction treatment is the discovery of the role of neuropeptides in addictive behaviors. Each emotion creates a unique neuropeptide, a chemical signature. Our cells become dependent on certain chemicals for survival, and as such, we literally become addicted to certain feeling states.

surrendering to one's suffering can bring about great change because the process of evolving is constant and held in a field of unconditional love that we all possess the ability to access.

Programs

Humans are very skilled at storytelling. It is how we process the world. Our stories live within us. Those of us with trauma histories are more likely to hold negative stories that inform our beliefs. A program is a set of internalized beliefs we interpret as true, and dictates how we think, feel, and behave. If you hold a core belief that you are not good enough—the classic toxic masculine program—then nothing you create will ever be good enough: you will never be good enough to receive love, you will never deserve to relax and feel joy, and so on. Programs are commonly held in the body, especially in the head, and are usually in opposition to the heart. Programs are internalized projections of the toxic masculine and are fear-based. They are connected to our egos, wounding, and intergenerational trauma. Many times, we are recapitulating programs handed down to us energetically through many generations. Programs are parts of us, but they are not real. For example, if you're running an old story that you'll be punished and abandoned if you speak your truth, you're running a program that no longer serves you. It is possible to discern what a program is, and what is real, what is fear-based, and what is rooted in love.

We have to hold space for our programs if we want to transform them. We are not here to be perfect, we are here to be human. This means holding space for all our parts. This does not mean covertly applying one's perfectionism onto the spiritual domain. What we resist persists, and so integrating all parts of ourselves unifies the whole. As Pema Chödrön says, "Nothing ever goes away until it has taught us everything we need to know."[20] We are so much more than the sum of our parts. We are not merely products of a clockwork universe, but multidimensional beings capable of infinite potentials.

When we recognize all our parts, we can witness our egos. Doing so gives us the power to exert more choice in our lives: in the systems we participate in, in the thoughts we entertain, and in the energies we engage. We are not our programs. Honoring our whole selves enables us to see where the ego is in the driver's seat and where the soul and our higher selves can come in to be in true co-creation. Flower essences are an amazing complement to deprogramming ourselves because they enhance the discernment process—we get to see what's truly part of our being, and what does not belong to us and can be let go.

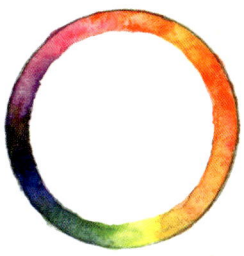

Return to Cosmic Balance

There was a time when we existed in a perfectly balanced state; all the natural world lived in harmony. Masculine and feminine held equal power in the cosmos. All the elements—earth, air, fire, and water—were in equilibrium. *Balance* is the operative word in many of the modalities with roots in the ancient healing traditions, such as Ayurveda, which asserts that optimal health is a result of balanced doshas; and traditional Chinese medicine (TCM), whose aim is to promote balance between all the elements and the yin (female) and yang (male). In the Egyptian mystery schools, initiates were expected to reach an internal position of balance in order to ascend to the next level. We all have the ability to reset our internal barometers to inner equilibrium.

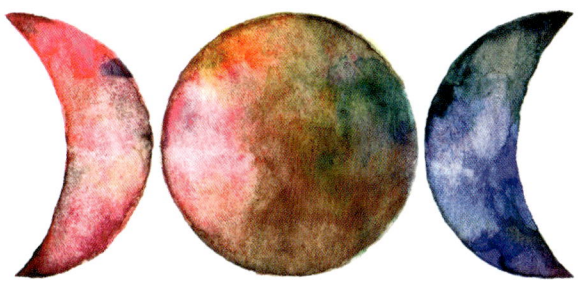

As humans, our beings hold a cellular memory of existing in a perfect state of wholeness, in unity consciousness. As our souls incarnated, we came into being from wholeness and grew into separation. Transpersonal psychologist Carl Jung conceived of a model of self that included:

- the ego—a small, mostly fear-based part of the self
- the conscious—what we know about ourselves
- the unconscious—what we don't know about ourselves, deep in the void

JUNG'S SYMBOL OF THE SELF

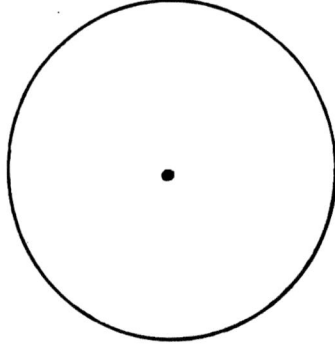

The concept of the *bio-psycho social-spiritual self,* or a multidimensional self, includes the dimensions of physical, mental, spiritual, community, and nature. I appreciate this model because it is inclusive and holistic. Who we are is so much more than our own limited thoughts and beliefs.

Energetically, we can look at how the chakras and personality develop as a way to understand how the self evolves. During childhood, the personality develops much like the physical body, and ego conflicts arise as a result of adapting to one's caregivers and environment. The energy systems grow in tandem with this process. Any imprinting during this time is usually the origin of many imbalances in the self. All of us have been imprinted with duality; this is the condition of being human.

In the human developmental process, a split occurs between our divine natures and our human natures. As we develop, parts of ourselves literally get left behind or

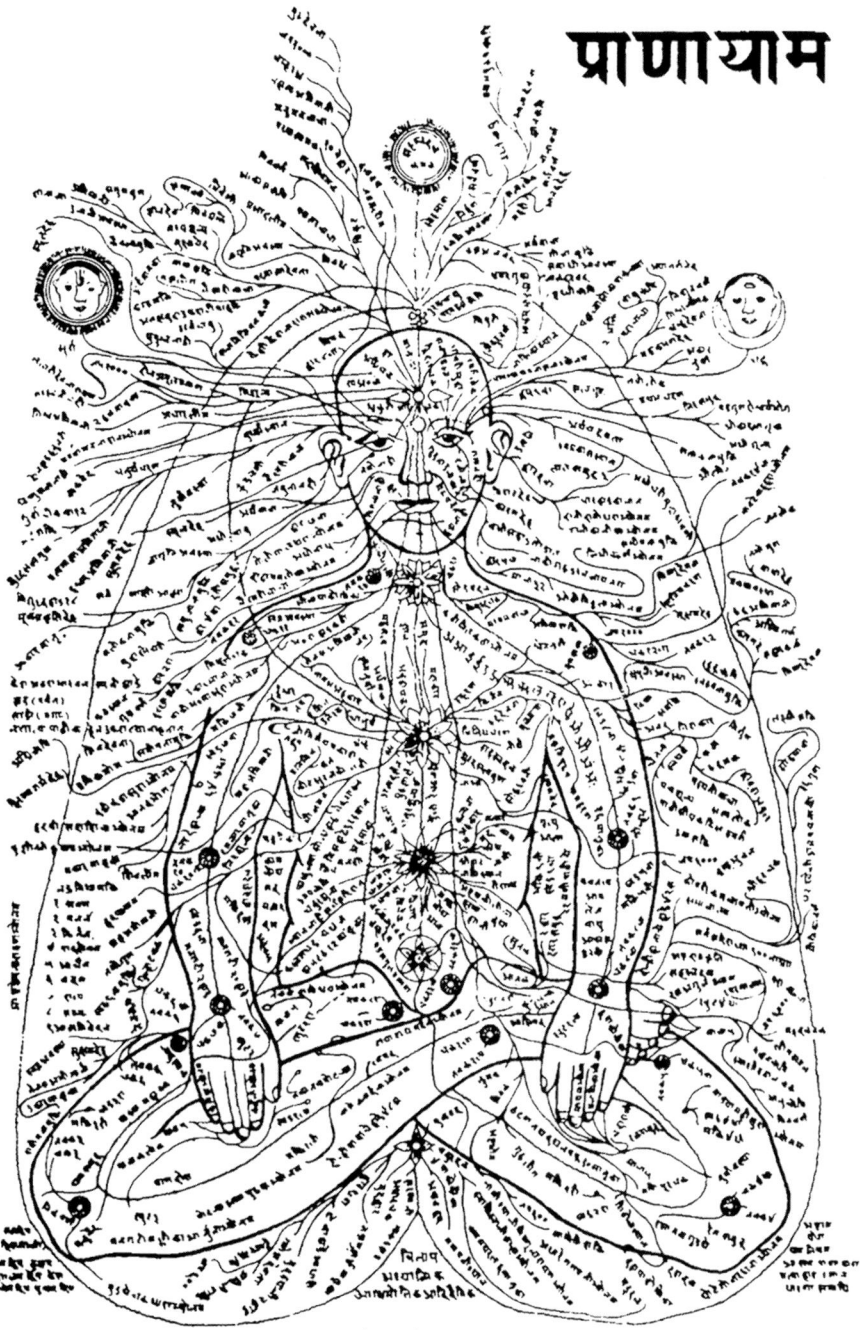

CHAKRA SYSTEM AND LESSER NADIS

frozen in time, a phenomenon addressed in soul retrieval work. The job of reintegration for some is very heavy work; some of us have deep trauma to heal. We all must integrate the parts of ourselves that went into duality. This is the root of all self-limiting beliefs and negative programs, and they almost always mirror characteristics of the toxic masculine.

Binary comparison or separation is one means of analysis. However, it is not possible to understand how plant medicine works solely by separating it into smaller and smaller parts and ignoring how the whole plant exists within its environment. Being human is similar: we are each a microcosm of the macrocosm of the Universe. In many holistic healing approaches, and especially in flower essence therapy, honoring the full spectrum of the human experience empowers us to feel more held and whole, in our experiences and in ourselves. Thinking in terms of either/or is limiting. Thinking in terms of both/and is expansive.

We free up so much energy when we are in this expanded state of awareness; it's a quantum way of being that aligns us more closely to co-creating with life instead of putting ourselves outside of it and looking in, separate from the world. Maya, in the Hindu tradition, is the illusion of separation that keeps us from being in harmony with the One, cut off from ourselves and source. Plants, in contrast, are in perfect relationship with nature. Plants—and being in right relationship with nature—show us how to honor our whole selves.

Choosing Conscious Beliefs

Our beliefs shape how we feel and function. We have been indoctrinated into belief systems of duality that denigrate the divine and the feminine, and this is the origin of much pathology and conflict on a collective level.

It's challenging to formulate an unbiased and healthy self-concept of ourselves if the beliefs that we've been programmed into are fear-based. The ego, associated with the mental body and the toxic masculine, usually has its own set of beliefs in opposition to that of the heart, which is associated with the soul. The wisdom and knowing of the soul/higher-self level is established by integrating the mind/masculine with the heart/soul—this is *discernment*. Everyone is free to believe whatever they like; this goes for both personal and general worldviews. However, if you choose what to believe without consciousness, out of fear, obedience to someone else, or reactively in rebellion, that is a problem. It's a problem because now every thought, emotion, and behavior that is attached to that belief system stems from fear rather than the truth. Much of what we believe about ourselves and reality has been coded into our major world religions and societal norms.

Many of the beliefs we hold were passed down intergenerationally. Every family has a set of rules based on ancestral beliefs, such as women should stay at home and men should earn a living. The collective also has a set of rules based on the cultural consciousness, such as women have no purpose in society after their childbearing years, or that the color of people's skin defines their worth. These rules are set up according to the needs of our family of origin and culture. It is the role we are asked to play to perpetuate the status quo, which is to say, to reinforce a largely patriarchal system. This is not about blaming our parents or our culture; it is about waking up to where we get to choose to participate in the cycle and make more conscious decisions.

Physical structures in our body resonate with our belief systems. So, if you were taught to believe, for example, that you were born in sin, and that you should be ashamed of your body, that will show up somewhere in your physical or subtle bodies. Or, going back to stress and relaxation, consider if your parents never took a vacation, perhaps because they needed to work all the time, which taught you that you should feel guilty about taking time off because they couldn't afford to. You've now unwittingly absorbed a family projection around relaxing.

We now know that multiple generations of genetic material are stored in our DNA, thus affecting how we function. Marginalized groups of extreme oppression, such as survivors of the Holocaust and descendants of slavery, hold a physiological inheritance of serious trauma.[21] The science of epigenetics, the study of how thoughts and emotions impact our genetic structures, further illustrates how what we believe affects us and our offspring on a cellular level.

As I've already shared, a collection of entrenched, unconscious beliefs is a program. A program is a crisis of consciousness. As children, we merge with our parents. We adopt much of their programming, which goes back for many, many generations. Many traumas and conflicts are passed down through multiple generations and lifetimes in order to be healed.* We absolutely have the opportunity to heal these programmed wounds, but it does require some work.

---

* The Flower Essence Society has a flower essence of Joshua tree for the very purpose of clearing intergenerational trauma.

At this point, with the aid of social media, we are waking up to many crises in consciousness on a massive scale. Socially, we are finally learning what it feels like to be a trans individual in America, what childhood looks like for a girl in a country controlled by religious extremists, and how dangerous it is to be black in the Midwest (and all parts of America). Environmentally, we are seeing the devastating effects that years of polluting our Earth are having on our water supply, and we are witnessing the extinction of so many of our precious animals. Politically, we are witnessing a time of great instability, where cameras and recorders are catching previously undocumented corruption. We are waking up to the realization that we are connected to all this—there is no separation—and accountability is shared by all. Waking up to our personal programs means waking up to it all.

Consciousness equals choice. This doesn't mean we get to control all the variables. Consciously choosing our beliefs gives us the ability to shape our thoughts, emotions, behavior, and overall well-being. It gives us the choice in how we live and how we feel. Many times, what we've been taught to believe is quite arbitrary, based on our family of origin and the place where we were born. While we don't get to control those factors, we do get to choose what is true.

Consciousness = Choice

CASE STUDY | Choosing Conscious Beliefs

Sam was a thirty-five-year-old American woman suffering from anxiety. The belief system she was raised within valued family, hard work, and obedience. She was also taught to believe that women should be subservient, that everything should appear "perfect" on the surface, and that you should never talk about your problems. Her father was occasionally physically abusive, and her mother was regularly emotionally and verbally abusive (she exhibited signs of both borderline and narcissistic personality traits). The abuse was covert, meaning that everyone assumed the family had no problems, but behind closed doors Sam lived in constant fear and confusion. She learned that this was normal behavior and assumed she deserved the treatment she received.

After running away at eighteen and paying her way through college, Sam excelled in her career and was able to buy a house. She exhibited tremendous resilience and agency. As we began our work together, we discovered that Sam held a lot of the beliefs about how she'd been treated as a child, and internalized them, believing at her core that she was bad and unworthy. She was unable to relax, felt a tremendous amount of guilt, and had trouble connecting intimately with others.

Culturally, the women in her lineage had suffered greatly, fleeing from one place to the next. Their only hope for survival was through marriage. Being a beautiful and agreeable woman was a top priority. In many ways, her family had been grooming her to become just like her mother: a disempowered, depressed woman whose only source of influence came through victimizing herself and making others feel guilty.

The other area we decided to address was Sam's fear of intimacy, which was connected to the hardening of herself as a child—a defense mechanism she employed to survive in her family. Because her parents had mistreated her, and she was not allowed to broach this subject with her parents (they needed to remain in denial), she was left to feel that she was bad and unlovable, that she deserved the mistreatment she suffered. This manifested in relationships with others that were ostensibly healthy, but lacked true affection and trust. Romantically, she attracted many emotionally unavailable partners.

By recognizing that there was a part of her that believed she didn't deserve love, she could see that this part was attached to her inner child, who was still scared (all parts of our inner child live inside us and retain their level of awareness unless we consciously work with them). By acknowledging her inner child, and validating her inner child's fears, she was able to move forward with confidence that she was, in fact, deserving and capable of giving and receiving love. Some of the essences that were vital to Sam's journey were that of ghost pipe to reconnect with divine love, pine to address the feelings of guilt, and golden amaranth to explore her relationship to relaxing.

Becoming more conscious is not a new concept—it's something we know how to do, we just have to remember how to do it! Becoming more conscious enables us to raise our vibration. Raising our vibration allows us to choose where we place our energy and to experience higher vibrational states of joy, beauty, gratitude, compassion, relaxation, and love. The moon reminds us that we are here to feel and allow all of human experience.

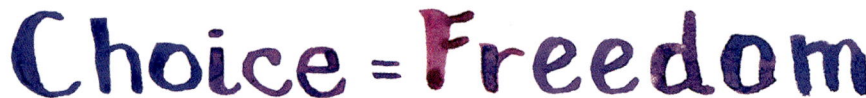

Focusing

Jane introduced me to the practice of Focusing—one of the most important tools in my spiritual toolbox. In the simplest terms, Focusing is about validating and spending time with your whole self—even and especially those parts you know and like the least. Of all the approaches I study, I always find myself coming back to Focusing. Why? Because it's simple, it's highly effective, it's not dogmatic, and it's a tool anyone can learn to use.

Focusing is a "body-oriented process of self-awareness and emotional healing" that involves "having a conversation with your feelings in which *you* do most of the listening.[22] By cultivating our *felt sense*, a subtle somatic awareness that arises in real time, we can access deeper states of knowing and healing. It's the most profound system for raising consciousness in the self that I have found. Developed by psychotherapist Eugene Gendlin, Focusing emerged from a collaboration with Carl Rogers, the founder of humanistic psychology. Ann Weiser Cornell, a linguist and former student of Gendlin, later expanded the theory to incorporate the ideas of presence, parts, neutrality, and the inner witness.[23]

In Focusing, we are asked to confront our inner duality, a polarity inherited, in my opinion, from the original cataclysmic masculine-feminine split. Unconsciously perceived as truth, we believe that parts of ourselves are bad. In order to heal ourselves, we believe these parts need to be denied, punished, cut off, released, and so on. This deeper exploration of our dualities is a perfect place to call on the gently uniting powers of flower essences. Echinacea is a wonderfully integrative flower essence to use while Focusing, as it assists us in making contact with parts of ourselves that may be less conscious.

When I explain Focusing to people, I like to use the metaphor of a house. We are like houses. The basement may be dirty or scary, the attic might be dangerous; we spend much time in some of the rooms, in others none at all. Focusing is like taking a candle into all the rooms and corners of the house, illuminating any areas that might be unconsciously or subconsciously causing us to experience a lower vibrational state (fear, sadness, shame, or anger), and showing us the way to bring light to those areas. The process is completely self-guided and natural, and engages both the physical and subtle bodies. Focusing informs all the rituals I explain later. The process of Focusing is so effective in large part because integrating on the soul level, uniting all our parts, is the natural state from which we evolved.

Can you be at peace with the parts that feel imperfect?

Is it possible to feel love for the parts of yourself you fear or dislike?

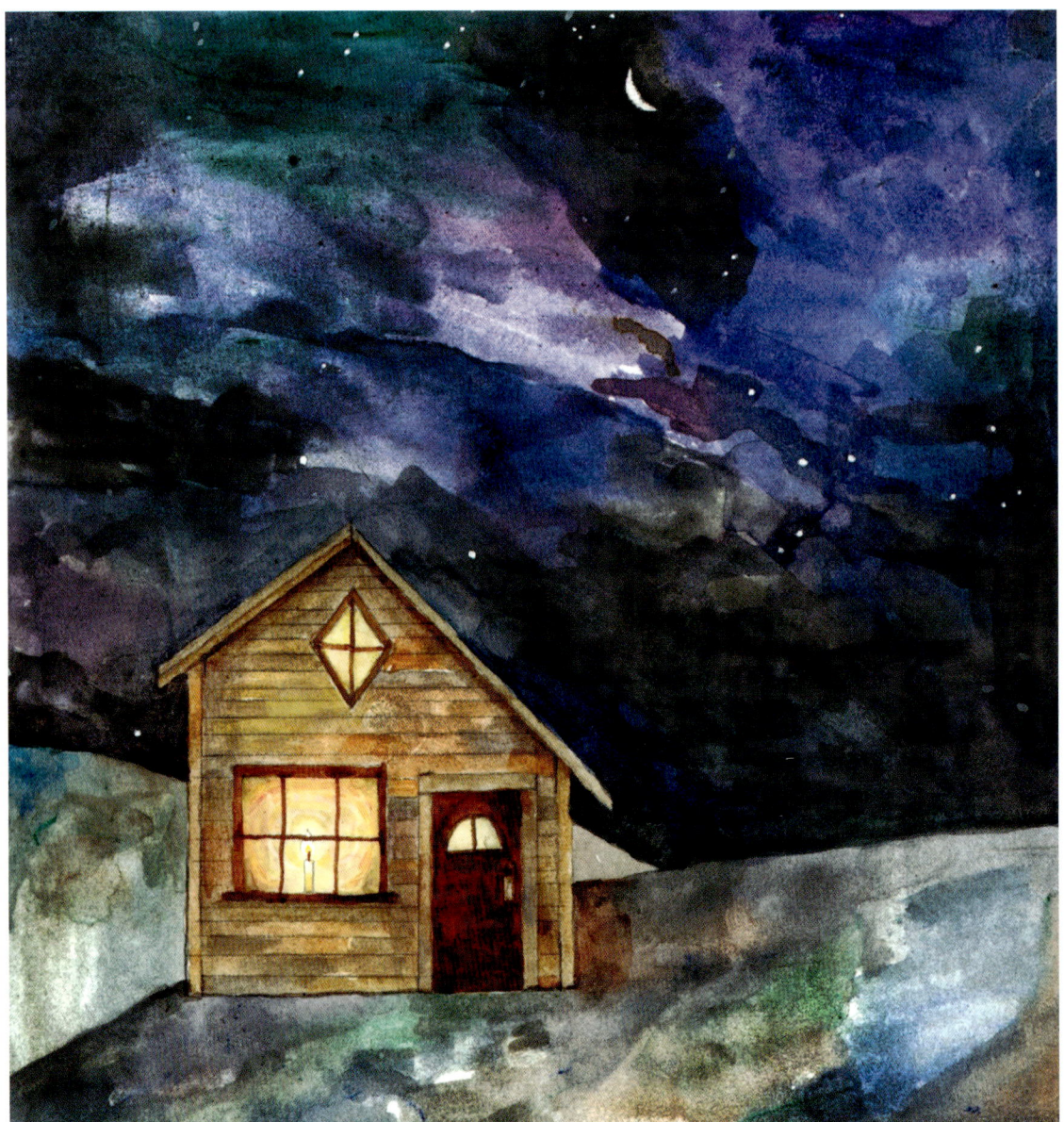

The Role of Relaxation

"Just relax." Sounds so simple, doesn't it? While we are wired for supreme relaxation, for many of us the modern nervous system is taxed and overstimulated. We need to rethink our relationship to relaxation and the role it plays in our lives. How you respond to stress informs a lot of your emotional and physical health. Most people who come to see me for help want to feel better, and a big part of this involves relaxing.

Everything runs more smoothly when we are in a relaxed state. We can access much more opportunity and higher vibrational states with more ease. We heal and age more optimally. We attract more grace. When we get out of our minds and relax into our bodies, true wisdom and intuition flow through us. There are so many flower essences that assist us in coming into deeper relaxation, and they are so effective, in part, because they show us where we are attached to negative or limiting beliefs about relaxing. All the remedies and modalities in the world won't make much of a difference if you are clinging to harmful beliefs about relaxing, such as "I don't deserve to feel good and relax" or "It doesn't feel safe to relax; I have to be busy all the time"—two very common programs I encounter.

We all have a survival consciousness encoded in our DNA. In the ancestral environment, we needed fear to motivate us as way to keep us alive. Now, the fears are somewhat different, but our reptilian brains are still part of us. Of course, there will be times when you are genuinely in survival mode, and you will need to function accordingly. But we all have a choice as to how much we want to engage the parts of ourselves that get activated in the face of stressful situations.

I often see people whose endocrine systems have been stressed to the point that they are basically in constant fight-or-flight mode: they exist the majority of the time in their sympathetic nervous system. The fear is perpetually turned "on," and the actual or perceived response is incongruent with reality; for example, their basic to-do lists give them panic attacks. I spent years in this place and know the toll it can take on a person. We reach this place because of our neurochemistry, how our caregivers modeled responding to stress, and how our culture impacts our stress response.

The respiratory system is the body system that can be consciously engaged most directly to affect the nervous system. Many of us have adopted breathing styles that activate our sympathetic nervous system, releasing stress hormones, including cortisol, which over time invites a host of health concerns, impairs a healthy stress response, and accelerates the aging process. Slowing the breath and bringing it down into the belly engages the parasympathetic nervous system (rest and digest), inhibits the production of stress hormones, and turns on our immune systems so we can heal. Deep breathing exercises are effective and work very well with flower essences. I've listed my top flower essences for relaxing in the next chapter.

Relaxing into Presence and Acceptance

Let's have a look at our relationship to time and the concept of presence. The modern world views time dualistically. We separate chronological time from eternal time. The Aboriginals viewed all time as past, present, and future as one, known as the Dreaming. Most ancient civilizations conceptualized time circularly, according to seasons and cycles. Conversely, our modern minds spend much of our time ruminating about the past and worrying about the future rather than existing in the present moment.

Becoming more present changed my life. In my twenties, I spent an inordinate amount of time busying myself, crossing things off lists, trying to control the future while simultaneously lamenting the past, believing that if I'd only "done it more perfectly back then," I would feel better now. Sound familiar?

Being present with yourself is foundational for healing work. If you want to go back and heal your past, you must hold space for the present, for everything that is showing up for you *now*. If you want to ascend into the higher vibratory states of love and bliss, you must come fully into the here and now to experience them. When you have more presence with yourself, you are able to be truly present with others, which is such a gift. Alan Watts described presence as the antidote to anxiety and suggested it was the one thing that separates us from the increasingly proliferate artificial intelligence.[24] With the advent of technology, many processes are quickening. (We even speed up natural processes like how fast livestock and plants grow, which is very detrimental to the Earth.) This attachment to speed and instant gratification pulls us out of natural cycles and the present. We can see the environmental metaphor of this as the seasons and weather patterns become increasingly unpredictable and volatile. I promise you that if you set an intention to be more present you will see and feel real change.

> *Radical Acceptance is the willingness to experience ourselves and our lives as it is.*
>
> TARA BRACH,
> *Radical Acceptance: Embracing Your Life With the Heart of a Buddha*

The negative polarity of acceptance is resistance, which uses up a lot of energy and keeps us from being present. Resisting our circumstances—how we feel, how others behave—isn't a good use of our energy and keeps us trapped in a victim mentality, separate from co-creating and vulnerable to the illusory external world. What I'm about to say may be very difficult for some people to hear, but I trust that we are ready as a collective to take responsibility for our trauma. Your wounds are your own to heal. No one else can do this work for you. If someone is a problem for you, that is your problem, not theirs. It is wonderful and wise to have a supportive healing circle around you, but the responsibility ultimately falls on you to accept and hopefully forgive. Similar to the act of surrender, acceptance is the process of taking accountability for your whole self and getting free from whatever is not you and not yours.

A lot of times in my work with people, we will come up against some resistance: to the self, to the process, to me, to a life situation. Resistance is always a doorway because it shows us where we are in resistance to our whole selves, or, not in acceptance of our whole selves. One way to resolve the duality of resistance is to simply ask: What am I resisting? or Where am I in resistance?

Flower essences create a safe container for this work to happen. Safety is of key importance in healing work because you cannot heal what you aren't ready to feel. This can be scary and is the main reason some choose to stay in duality and unconsciousness.

Frequently, I will observe a progression from less conscious states (associated with lower vibrational states) to more conscious states (associated with higher vibrational states). This is not to say that we don't suffer as we become more conscious! If we are truly open to the process of awakening, then we have to let go of wanting to control what doorways present themselves. Presence and acceptance allow us to move beyond over-attachment to feeling states in general, and simply into being. Believing that we should always feel good, or that something is always wrong, actually constitutes resistance (the opposite of acceptance) in disguise. Sound healer Tom Kenyon feels that the way we evolve and become more conscious occurs dramatically when we exist in states of compassion and appreciation, a process he calls *upleveling*.[25] Some feel upleveling is the process of moving out of 3-D consciousness into more expanded 4-D and 5-D consciousness.

Presence~Acceptance~Gratitude

Radical Self-Care

Attending to our personal needs from a place of self-love and compassion is not something that is built into our Western cultural education. It's counter to what we've been taught, which is that care should take place outside of oneself, if at all. We are taught to put the needs of others before our own, which is especially the case for women—caring for oneself implies a weakness and vulnerability; it's only accessible to wealthy, white folks, and the like. The shadowy side of self-care would be the dimension that has been co-opted and commodified toward overindulgence and bypassing, or worse yet, a perpetuation of privilege onto marginalized groups.

I consider self-care to be truly taking care of yourself for the betterment of all. It's essential to remember two things when discussing self-care: 1) self-care should be in the service of self-love; and 2) it should be understood that caring for oneself is synonymous with caring for one's community and the Earth, because there is no separation between inner and outer work. Yes, self-care is imbued with much privilege, and not everyone has access to getting a massage, or is in a financial situation that would allow them to leave a toxic relationship to focus on themselves. And, we need to take care of ourselves in all the ways that we are able. Understanding the interconnectedness of caring for yourself and doing it from a loving place of devotion is what makes self-care radical.

We can't do all the work of waking up and healing unless we are caring for ourselves. It's not getting easier to exist on our planet. The cost of living has skyrocketed. We are contending with greater social, economic, political, and environmental instability. While a lot of the old oppressive structures are coming into question and collapsing, the fallout from this creates a lot of stress for us to manage. We are doing our best to raise the next generation to cope with accelerated volatility and looming catastrophes. It's not a particularly positive or pleasant time to be human (or plant or animal, sadly) in many ways. To balance all these factors, we must take extra care of ourselves and each other. The rules of existing on this planet have changed, and more is simply required for us to survive and thrive.

If trauma lives at one side of a polarity, resilience occupies the other side. Resilience is the ability to adapt in times of conflict. There are times when we need to draw from our personal banks. Building up our resilience can support us when we are running at a deficit. As we open, grow, and heal, we are able to tolerate a wider spectrum of the human experience, to welcome it all. The natural world is full of resilience, and adapting to one's environment amid stress is the evolutionary process. Humans are tremendously resilient beings, and caring for ourselves and our communities magnifies our collective potential.

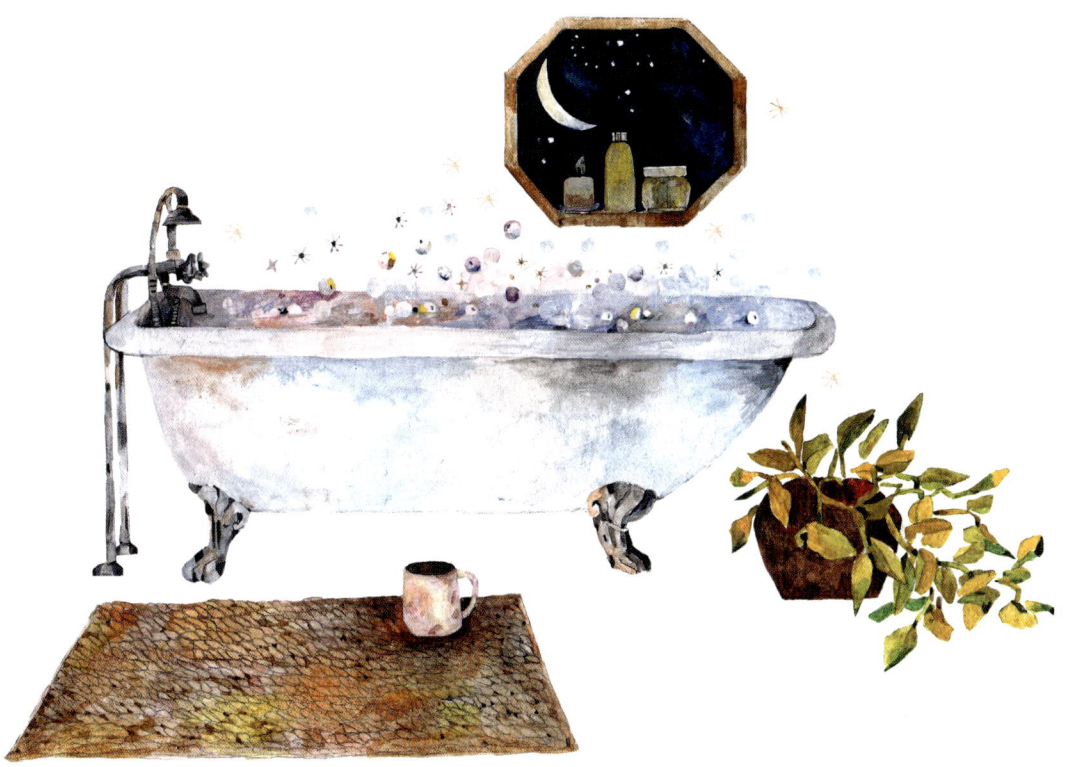

Flower essences generally attract empaths, people who are very sensitive to their environments and the energies of others. Empaths care deeply for all life because they *feel* all life deeply. Empaths need to be extra careful of their energy because they can be more vulnerable to sickness and burnout. Change makers, activists, helpers of all kinds must take extra care because the demand for change and collective healing is not slowing, it is only growing.[26] Related to this is the concept of healthy boundaries.

Having healthy boundaries means caring for yourself by being discerning of where you invest your energy, and when you say yes and no. The feminine embodies nurturance and compassion. The empowered feminine is fiercely protective of itself, its loved ones, and its convictions. The divine feminine knows exactly when and how to say no. Healer and sacred sexual teacher Juliet Haines says that one says no from the second chakra, from the sex organs.[27] Often, self-care means saying no: to a toxic relationship, an obligation, a negative thought loop, and so forth. When you say no to something that is not nourishing to you, you can then draw the energy that was leaking in that space of your life and redirect it inward to care for yourself.

Flower essences make a beautiful complement to any self-care regimen. In fact, one of my favorite essences to support self-care is self-heal. Essences can be used alone or in a group setting. Some ways flower essences can be incorporated into self-care are:

- making a special flower essence blend to add to a bubble bath
- taking a grounding tree essence such as redwood or pine and then going for a walk in the woods
- offering a protective essence for a group moon ceremony or supportive gathering
- making medicine with a nervine plant, such as chamomile or lavender, as a group to gift to others for self-care

Again, self-care can't be just about caring for ourselves, because we don't heal in a vacuum, we heal together. Who we are is connected to our ancestors, community, and nature. The mind-body-spirit movement is booming, and we can't become complacent here. We must keep exploring how self-care spaces, such as yoga studios and healing collectives, can become more inclusive and accessible.[28] Remember, none of us heal unless we all heal. The greater capacity you have to love yourself, the greater capacity you can give.

Being of Service

The ancients held such a profound respect for life that it translated into a solid balance between all living things and the understanding that all were interconnected in the ascension process. Hopefully, in your evolution, you will find a balance in your relationship to being of service. Either you will recognize needs beyond your own, or you will prioritize your own needs, or both. Being of service doesn't mean abandoning your own needs, but rather recognizing how your healing creates quantum healing and abundance. It also doesn't mean taking on the responsibility to heal others—that is codependence. When you become aware of how to discern what is of service to your soul as opposed to your ego, you will attract more grace and opportunity into your life and invite more light to flow through you. Some of us have been given tremendous gifts in our lifetime, and therefore, we have the opportunity to give back in big ways. To those that much has been given, much can be shared.

Pursuant to presence, a recent study by Loretta Pyles concluded that being in service increases one's "subjective sense of having a lot of time."[29] A common misconception connected to egoic consciousness is that there is only so much abundance to go around. The "what's in it for me" mentality is embedded in most of our economic structures. Only looking out for yourself keeps you trapped in the 3-D, separated from your true self, your authentic connection with others, and source. Nurturing, mothering, and supporting are all service virtues of the feminine domain.

Beyond what we have to offer materially, we always have the opportunity to be generous in spirit. Generosity is a giving energy from the heart, while attachment is a holding energy away from the heart.[30]

True giving is a thoroughly joyous thing to do. We experience happiness when we form the intention to give, in the actual act of giving, and in the recollection of the fact that we have given. Generosity is a celebration.

SHARON SALZBERG

It is a natural phenomenon that when you begin working with flower essences you will become more aware in general: of the natural world, of other people's experiences, of the suffering of the animal kingdom and the Earth. This is because, as I've mentioned, the flowers engage the heart, and the heart is what connects us to nature. You may feel more pain as a result of this boost in awareness, and you will also be gifted with more energy with which to serve. Even if you didn't have it before, you will be given what you need to be of service, because you are tapped into universal consciousness, the heartbeat of the Earth. The Universe cannot run out of energy—it's infinite.

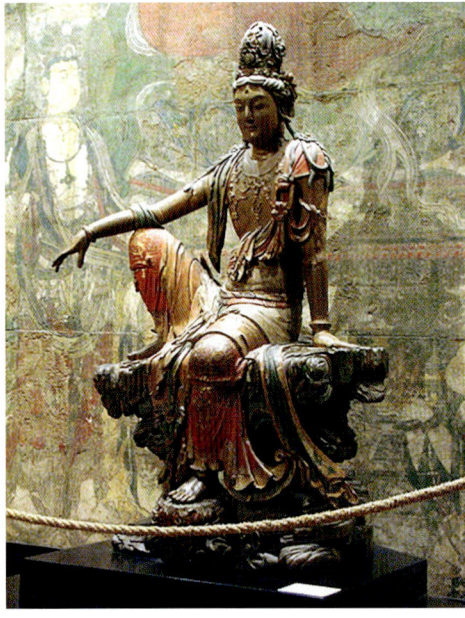

THE BODHISATTVA GUANYIN (KUAN YIN), Goddess of Compassion (eleventh–twelfth century, northern China). Bodhisattvas are beings who have decided to incarnate to help others, despite having reached nirvana. Before Siddhartha Gautama became Buddha, he was a bodhisattva. Photo by Rebecca Arnett.

Healing for Ourselves, the Collective, and the Planet

When you open yourself up to the plant kingdom, new awareness can develop. You can become more empathic, which sounds pleasant in theory, but can be overwhelming because now you're not just experiencing more of your own feelings, but the feelings of others as well. If you're committed to applying a healing justice framework in your work, you will likely expose new trauma and have to reckon with your own privilege, which can be painful. You could develop more attunement with nature, which also can feel wonderful and, because of the tragic state of our Earth, completely disorienting. At this time, we are experiencing a heightened polarity between the light and the dark. We are being asked to hold a neutral space for all this duality and to have more compassion for all life. Flower essences enhance the energetic interconnection between all living things and so are especially well suited to support an expansion of consciousness.

Understanding how we function within—and our responsibility to—the collective is important because none of us operates alone. If you forget what you derive from the collective, you assume you don't owe it anything and exist separately from everyone. Much of the privileged world enjoys the benefits of being part of the collective, whether we are conscious of it or not: rights, amenities, protection, accessible health care, clean drinking water, electricity, and so on. So, those with the material upper hand at this time have a special responsibility to the rest of those sharing the Earth. We are all dependent on one another to collectively wake up and heal.

At this point in time, we are being asked to go beyond the limited, narcissistic view of the self and open ourselves to the self in connection with our environment. This is our exalted self. Just like the plant kingdom, we need to be in balance with each other and our entire environment in order to survive and thrive.

The next Buddha will be the sangha.

THICH NHAT HANH

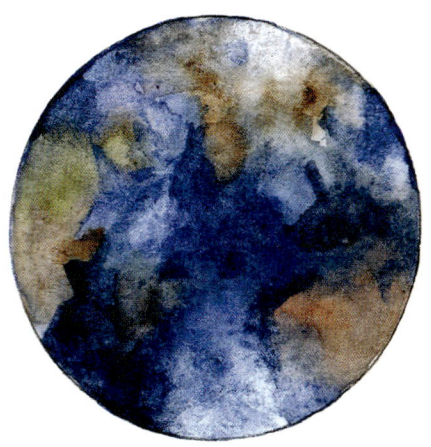

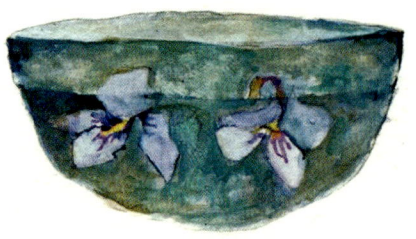

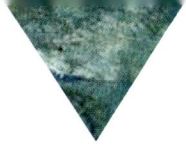

CHAPTER THREE

The Blooms

THESE ARE CHAOTIC TIMES, and yet the laws of nature support all life coming into balance. We, too, have tremendous opportunities to come into greater equilibrium by balancing the duality within ourselves, and to live in greater heart consciousness. Inner disharmony is something that Dr. Bach understood as the true origin of emotional and physical disease. Coming into right relationship with ourselves includes how we are in relationship with our environment. In the previous chapter, we looked at some various ways of coming into cosmic balance, and this chapter will expand on how flower essences can be used in the service of this evolution.

Plant and vibrational medicines are the oldest forms of healing on the planet, connected to much ancient wisdom that is crucial for us to remember now. These primordial precepts have many analogs with emerging quantum theory that can be applied to understanding flower essences, which I will share by highlighting more information around vibrational, or subtle, energetic medicine. When we talk about ancient plant wisdom and healing traditions, we are borrowing from many cultures and should be sensitive to amalgamating this information for our own use. Pursuant to this, it's time we apply more social and healing justice considerations to all healing modalities, including flower essences. A social and healing justice model is a holistic and inclusive framework that essentially incorporates the impact of duality and oppression on us: mind, body, and soul, with the aim of liberating us all.

Defining flower essences requires some imagination because no universal definition exists. They aren't exactly things—they are more of a process. The word *flower* actually derives from the word *flowing*. In describing what flower essences are—how and why they work, how they've come to exist, how to understand their significance and application—it's possible to conceptualize them as falling under two therapeutic subsets: herbal medicine and vibrational medicine. Flower essences are physical remedies you take orally (or apply topically) that are made by harnessing the subtle energies of a flower. They are a wondrous blend of herbal and vibrational medicine that can lead to transformations beyond what your current consciousness may even believe is possible.

My interpretation of flower essences is based on formal study, clinical practice, and my own personal experience. It is subjective, as is an analysis of any healing modality. I am also writing from the perspective of a white, middle-class, cisgender woman of European descent. I have bias and am a recipient of much privilege, for instance being in a position to write this book. I am also committed to the continual inquiry around where my interpretations and practice may be unconsciously perpetuating this bias and privilege. In comparing the literature, I've sought to honor the work of those who have come before me, as well as shed light on the disproportional influence of Euro-American men in herbal medicine and the origins of flower essence therapy. While producers and practitioners will use different lenses to explain flower essences, we all seek to understand the truth in order to use the essences for the greater good of people and the planet. The social and healing justice movements have affected me deeply, and it is my sincere hope that we can continue to decolonize and dismantle where dominant systems are limiting the positive proliferation of alternative healing and flower essence therapy to make them more accessible and inclusive. The more we come into balance in this way, the more transformation is available to us all, our communities, and our Earth. And the more we maintain plant medicine as medicine for all people.

I feel called to frame the study of flower essences within the disciplines of herbal medicine and vibrational medicine because these two subsets most closely encompass what flower essences are. Vibrational medicine, sometimes also called subtle energetic medicine, uses specialized forms of energy to positively affect those energetic systems that may be out of balance due to disease states. Additionally, we need to expand this definition to clarify that "energy" can either be physical or subtle (e.g., plant medicine or flower essence), or both. It is the life force, vitality, or energy that connects all life. Herbalism, or plant medicine, is the practice of the medicinal and therapeutic use of plants to support health and wellness. Herbalism also directly connects us with the macrocosm.

Vibrational medicine and herbalism share a number of similarities, including:

- encouraging balance to facilitate greater states of healing
- emphasizing healing from levels within the self, as well as harmonizing the mind-body-spirit connection
- seeking to do no harm (as the ancient Greek Asclepius of Thessaly is credited with saying: "first the word, then the plant, then the knife")
- engaging the subtle bodies (emotional, mental, astral, and physical)
- connecting us with the Earth and the other kingdoms (plant, mineral, and animal)
- being types of alternative health approaches/complementary and alternative medicine (CAM)
- being informed by ancient and indigenous wisdom

Within a more Western nomenclature, flower essences are considered a type of herbal CAM. The World Health Organization (WHO) defines herbal medicine to "include herbs, herbal materials, herbal preparations and finished herbal products, that contain as active ingredients parts of plants, or other plant materials, or combinations,"[1] and flower essences would fall into this category. The National Center for Complementary and Integrative Health (NCCIH), which was formed by the National Institutes of Health (NIH) and funds research and clinical trials of CAM techniques, does not currently include flower essences in its areas of research.[2] However, systems such as TCM, Ayurveda, naturopathy, herbalism, homeopathy, and energy therapies such as qigong and Reiki are included. According to the NCCIH, "If a non-mainstream practice is used together with conventional medicine, it's considered 'complementary'" and "if a non-mainstream practice is used in place of conventional medicine, it's considered 'alternative.'"[3] Integrative medicine is considered to be conventional and complementary approaches together. Functional medicine is also a term that is increasingly used to describe integrative approaches of healing.

The tension between sun and moon consciousness extends into Western medicine, where it presents as the seemingly oppositional argument between reductionist, mechanical (masculine) and holistic (feminine) philosophies. However, integrating these two ideologies allows us to understand both the parts and the whole system. There is a place for empiricism as well as qualitative and phenomenological analysis in flower essence therapy. Both are valid; both sides are necessary for seeing the flowers' potential. At the levels of wave function and quantum entanglement, everything in our cosmos is connected, regardless of time or space.

Plant medicine exists on a spectrum of Western and empirical on one end, and very spiritual and abstract on the other. Flower essences serve as a bridge between the two orientations. Throughout history, many Western herbalists have spoken to the efficacy of an "energetic" or "homeopathic" dose of herbs taken in one- to two-drop dosages, and so the vibrational, or energetic, application of herbs has probably always been in use. Machaelle Small Wright of Perelandra has opened up what she calls her "co-creative relationship with nature" intelligences to include an impressive system of working with the spirit realm. The Flower Essence Society has gained much validation from the scientific community through its clinical studies, and David Dalton of Delta Gardens uses his flower essences to address both the physical as well as the psycho-spiritual. The applications of flower essence therapy are as manifold and as unique as the individuals who utilize them.

Herbal and vibrational medicines are united in their goal of bringing the individual (and, by proxy, the Earth) into balance. Because we're working with natural forces—and nature inherently finds balance since this is the state in which all life proliferates—the balancing of all energies is of great significance. True balance occurs when we are in alignment with our highest selves, beyond the level of the ego. This means we have reached a place of connection with our hearts and the Earth. My goals as a practitioner are always to promote the spirit of opening and living in the heart. Taking and making flower essences are in supreme service of this objective.

This chapter serves as a basic framework to understand how flower essences work and how to use them in practice. I have endeavored to further explain the system of vibrational medicine to clarify misconceptions and offer new insight into this theory of healing. Working with flower essences is a highly subjective art form, but objective patterns can be observed in the application of the remedies. It's a very creative endeavor to design your own healing practice, whether for your own individual use or in a professional practice helping others. You get to decide how and what informs your approach.

A NOTE ABOUT SEXUALITY AND NATURE

In this book, I am very interested in the masculine and feminine. I acknowledge that the terms "masculine" and "feminine" do not resonate with all people. It is not my intention to perpetuate the problematic binary system and heteronormativity within the healing process. There is much allusion to masculine and feminine in nature. Nature is very bisexual, hermaphroditic, and diverse. Likewise, energy has many dimensions: it can be masculine, feminine, both, or neither.

What Are Flower Essences?

The National Institutes of Health defines flower essences as an "alternative health approach." Practitioners will define flower essences in different ways. When dealing with the subtle realms, subjectivity abounds. I prefer the description offered by Gurudas, who wrote one of the early books on flower essences and vibrational healing with the help of a gifted channel. He defines them as

> *tinctures of liquid consciousness, and stored within them is an evolutionary force, the life force itself shaped to a particular pattern depending on the signature of the particular plant and/or flower. This liquid consciousness can be considered educational for the psychospiritual dynamics of an individual. Working with these vibrations offers one an opportunity to shift one's beliefs, conceptions, ideas of science, and long-term patterns to a place of greater awareness and understanding.*[*][4]

The following are some of the ways flower essences are defined (taken from producers' websites).

---

[*] Gurudas is understood as a controversial figure within the flower essence community. While I don't subscribe to his theories unequivocally, I do think there is a place for his contributions to flower essence therapy, especially as they relate to our understanding of vibrational medicine and energy.

The Perelandra essences are oral solutions taken to balance and stabilize the body's electric system and its circuits. They are also taken for maintaining the overall strength and balance in the electric system.

—Machaelle Small Wright [5]

The role of flower essences is to assist humanity to clear emotional or astral bodies of those conditions that pre-dispose them to disease.... Flowers are the highest manifestation of the life force of the plant.

—Findhorn Essences [6]

Flower essences are liberating in that they enable us to see through restrictive conditionings and belief systems imposed by our respective cultures. They do this in an unobtrusive manner. They assist by catalyzing expansion rather than forcing it.

—Luminesce, producer of Living Light Essences
and distributor or Bloesem Remedies Nederland [7]

How Flower Essences Work

Both plant medicine and vibrational medicine aim to bring the body into balance by supporting the whole individual: the physical, emotional, and spiritual. Plant and vibrational medicines connect us to our ancestors and help us to come into greater harmony with our environment. They can also be applied to plants and animals, and are not bound by time or space. Like with any medicine, we can observe how flower essences function based on the effects they produce within us and within our environments. Flower essences contain no physical plant constituents; rather, the vibrational signature of the plant is energetically extracted into a remedy.[8]

Flower essences are created from blossoms that have been picked at the height of their blooms, placed in a solution of water that has been charged by the sun, and preserved in a small amount of alcohol. Their special relationship to the light is a part of their unique healing properties. Each essence contains the energetic template of that plant, which is then overlaid on our crystalline matrix to bring in more light. Author and flower essence practitioner Julian Barnard writes that "Dr. Bach's flower remedies are centrally concerned with bringing light to the light body," and that "the flower essence becomes a vehicle for preserving and transferring this light resonance to another person in another place."[9]

About half of Bach's essences are produced via the boiling method, wherein the heartier plants such as pine and willow are first gently simmered in boiling water for thirty minutes, then prepared just as those via the sun method.

Flower essences are different from essential oils and are odorless. The entire signature—or essence—of the flower is captured in the medicine. The flower essence tincture can be taken orally, applied directly to the skin, or made into a mist. They are safe, nontoxic, and have no side effects. They are appropriate for use with adults, children, animals, and plants.

What Does Energetic Mean?

What exactly is meant by the term *energetic* in the context of plant medicine and flower essences? In addition to their physical signature (such as the shape or color of a plant), flower essences work on subtle energetic or vibrational levels, and possess an energetic signature. Patricia Kaminski calls this a "numinous quality."[10] The state or situation to be addressed is also energetic (such as a heavy, stagnant depression). Plants (and stones) hold the energetic memory of our earliest existence. They evolved with us and carry information to help us heal. Every plant has a vibrational signature, an adaptation or gesture of how the plant exists in relation to its environment. This presentation alludes to its healing properties and can be thought of as the plant's personality. For example, the way in which a morning glory opens toward the light and closes at night illustrates its efficacy as a flower essence in addressing diurnal cycles. The energetic signature can be visible, as in the case of the action of the morning glory. It can also be more subtly perceived; for instance, the way ghost pipe connects one to divine love, or marshmallow can be used to soften one's heart. Plants have a light body, or subtle body, just as humans do.

A plant's energetics are connected to its actions, which are similar to tissue states: hot, cold, dry, damp, constriction, relaxation. Some practitioners within Ayurveda and TCM work from a list of twenty energetic qualities.[11] Karyn Sanders is an herbalist with whom I've had the privilege of studying, whose work is based in Native American energetic herbalism. According to Sanders, illness is caused when energy either becomes static or dissipates, and we must be able to see what a balanced state for ourselves (or client) looks like. Sanders also feels that the idea of directional energy is very important to consider, otherwise you could be making an issue worse.[12] Some examples of energetics would be

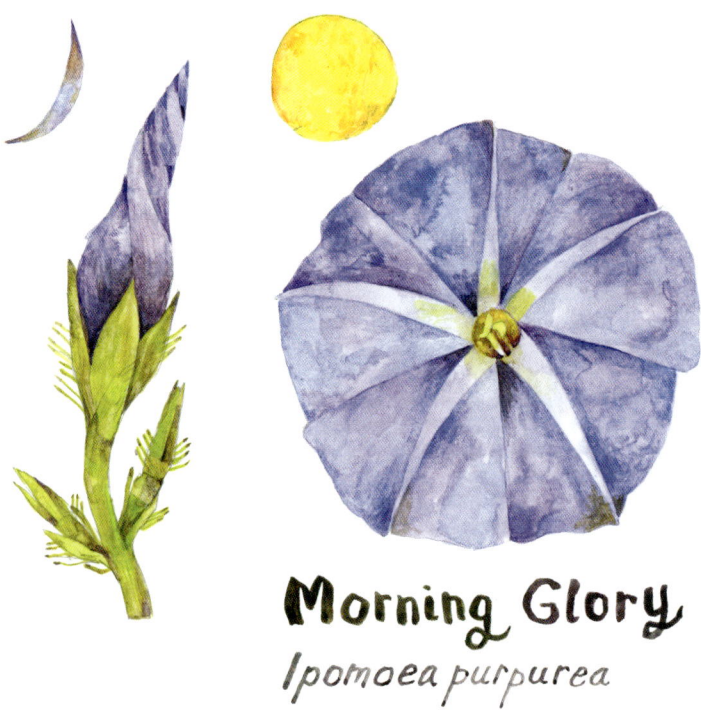

Morning Glory
Ipomoea purpurea

grounding, moving, warming, dispersing, and cooling. Energetics can also be experienced even more abstractly, such as through the nurturing, maternal energy of the madrone tree. By working energetically with a plant, we can match its energy with that of a condition and a person's constitution or baseline functioning.

The way I work with energy and energetics is with the felt sensations and inner knowing that arise within me when working with a person and/or a plant. It is different than checking a box in a physical assessment. I am relying on the information or wisdom to pass through me, then I observe it. In this way, I am allowing the person/or plant to guide what is coming into the field to be addressed. I'm not so much directing this process as I am holding a container for it. For instance, if someone is experiencing a lot of anxiety as a result of an upcoming public speaking engagement, and I know this person tends to dissociate or go out of their body when nervous, I will include an essence such as oak to help them stay in their body and root into the Earth to counterbalance the up-and-out energy.

The art of subtle perception, intuition, and working with energy was the way of the ancients and is connected to many indigenous healing traditions still practiced today by various groups throughout the world. Quantum physics will continue to validate ideas around energy as it challenges our traditional understandings of time, space, and dimensional reality. Quantum physics' and energetic applications to science and medicine are in progress, and working energetically is a vital and valid way to engage in healing work.

Like many vibrational or subtle energetic modalities, flower essences work with the chakra system. During childhood, as the personality develops, ego conflicts arise as a result of adapting to our caregivers and environment. The energy systems develop in tandem with this process. Any imprinting during this time is usually the origin of many imbalances in the system. Left unaddressed, psycho-spiritual conflicts in our unconscious and subconscious can become full-blown mental and physical conditions. Imbalances are always healing opportunities. Flower essence therapy aims to expand our awareness of how early and ongoing conditions are informing present issues, and to enable healing, integration, and release.

The goals of flower essence therapy include: ease in accessing higher vibratory states like joy and gratitude; enhanced mind-body-spirit balance, presence, acceptance of emotions and integration of difficult vibratory states; encouraging flow states like creativity; manifesting; supporting balance; expanding awareness of self and the Universe, ancestral connection and healing; and helping us to be of greater service to ourselves, others, and the Earth.

Flower essences work by way of the following:

- synchronicities—helping us connect seemingly unrelated or previously unseen opportunities or happenings
- indirect occurrences—positively affecting different environments and interpersonal dynamics
- insights—supporting mental, emotional, physical, and/or astral awakening; new ideas, solutions, or information may present
- physical changes—bringing up new sensations, shifts in organ/system functioning or in symptoms
- emotional responses—bringing up new feelings or memories; stabilizing or releasing them
- expression—inspiring artistic, verbal, and kinesthetic expression

- dreamtime—bringing about new or recurring dreams, insights, and subconscious resolution
- invoking intention—the more time and space you can offer, the more likely you'll be able to feel flower essences. For example, taking them with a light meditation, a visualization, while doing yoga or some other kind of bodywork or prayer

CASE STUDY | Synchronicity in the Healing Process

The more I work with flower essences, the more I am constantly amazed at the way they heal. In the beginning of my practice, I still held some skepticism connected to my rational mind. While my intention was to be a clear vessel for light to pass through to my clients, I'm sure the vibrational imprint of my doubt colored that intention to some extent. Despite this, my clients would connect with the essences and feel the effects.

Several years later, I was working with a young woman who had recently suffered the loss of her mother. The young woman had a collection of healers and doctors she regularly saw for support. She came to me as a last resort (I get quite a few of these clients). She had been operating in survival mode for most of her life and was presenting with symptoms of serious anxiety, depression, gastritis, and adrenal fatigue. When I suggested that I felt the underlying cause of her symptoms was connected to not having let herself grieve the loss of her mother, she broke down in tears, which confirmed my intuition.

I gave her a blend of olive for exhaustion, motherwort for the dependency she still felt for her mother, and borage for her heavy heart. I felt confident that this blend would help her. Her guides had been very clear with me when I formulated it. And though she had felt deeply seen and validated in our last session, when I gave the tincture to her, she held the bottle and hunched over in her chair. "You don't believe this will help?" I asked. She gave pause, then said, "No, I guess I don't. Not after all the other stuff I've been doing that hasn't worked." So we spent a few minutes with the part of herself that believed she shouldn't feel better because her mother was gone. This part also believed it would lose a connection to her mother if she improved (a persistent pattern when her mother was alive). She was able to name these connections and began to see roses everywhere when taking the tincture. They reminded her of her mother, and a different connection opened for her there. (We would later include rose in another blend that was also very effective.) After a few days, she reported feeling a warm, suffusing energy around her shoulders and heart. She said she began to feel hopeful about the year ahead.

    I offer this story to illustrate two points. First, the flower essences will work regardless of whether or not you believe they will be effective. However, their potency will be enhanced if you trust in their efficacy. And the best way to truly know this is to spend some time with the flowers. Secondly, the synchronicity of the roses may or may not have correlated with taking the essence, but I don't feel my client would have connected seeing the roses to her mother had she not been taking that particular blend. She said that she felt that the tincture widened the scope of her vision to receive healing from other places she wouldn't have been open to seeing otherwise.

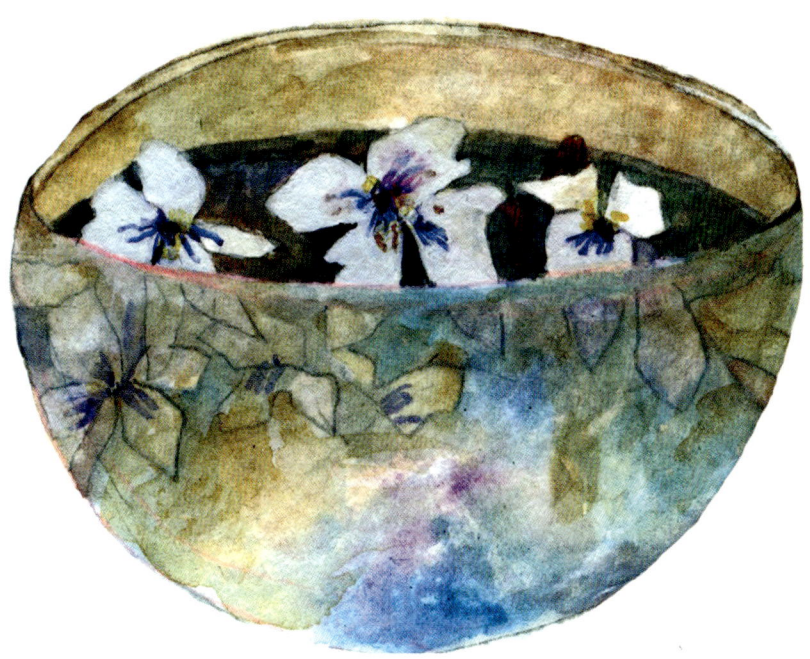

IS MY FLOWER ESSENCE WORKING?

Flower essences can work on both subtle and physical levels. Sometimes they are working in ways that are beyond our waking consciousness. Every experience with flower essences is unique to each individual because we are working with the alchemy of science and spirit (as opposed to inert synthetic chemicals with very controlled outcomes). The more open you are to the process, and the more time and space you allow the flower essences to work, the more likely you will connect with them. Sometimes it's helpful to work with a flower essence practitioner to assess how you are responding to your remedy.

Herbal Medicine

Herbal medicine is also referred to as herbalism, plant medicine, phytology, and botanical or biomedicine. It is the use of plants for medicinal use. Food is also considered medicine in this context. A Western shamanic branch of herbalism is sometimes known as plant spirit medicine, as coined by herbalist Eliot Cowan, and emphasizes journeying with the plant spirits and elementals. All ancient civilizations utilized plants as medicine, and modern herbalism is informed by traditions from all over the world. One of the earliest known instances of plant medicine is that of a "flower burial" of a Neanderthal in a cave in Iraq, dating to approximately 50,000 years ago.[13] Ayurvedic medicine can be found in the Vedas, sacred Hindu texts, and the practice dates back to approximately 7,000 BCE to the Indus Valley.[14] Ancient Egyptian medicine was a highly sophisticated system that included extensive written record of herbal (and animal) treatments and diagnoses for each body system, including many surgical interventions as far back as 4,500 BCE. Many physicians of this time period were also priests and scribes. Ancient Egyptian medicine largely influenced the Greek humoral tradition that would go on to serve as the foundation for Western herbalism, although the Egyptian contribution is not usually acknowledged. Traditional Chinese and Tibetan medicines were practiced in Asia as far back as 1,400 BCE and featured a specific relationship between the body's meridians (energetic channels) and plants.[15]

Within the Western tradition, plants' healing properties are conveyed via their "doctrine of signature"; that is, the way in which the plant has adapted to its environment and assumes certain forms. A signature is a collection of characteristics about a plant that offers us clues as to how the plant works, and how we can work with it. In the plant spirit medicine tradition, plants can speak to us through the elements—earth, air, fire, water (wood and metal too), through our dreams, other nature spirits, and our ancestors. As we already discussed, plants have an energetic signature as well, and this is especially true for flower essences.

Take *Aloe vera* (*Aloe barbadensis*), for instance. Aloe is used herbally as a treatment for skin conditions and to soothe the epithelial lining of our digestive systems. Its actions are cooling and moisturizing. If you've ever touched an aloe leaf, you'll

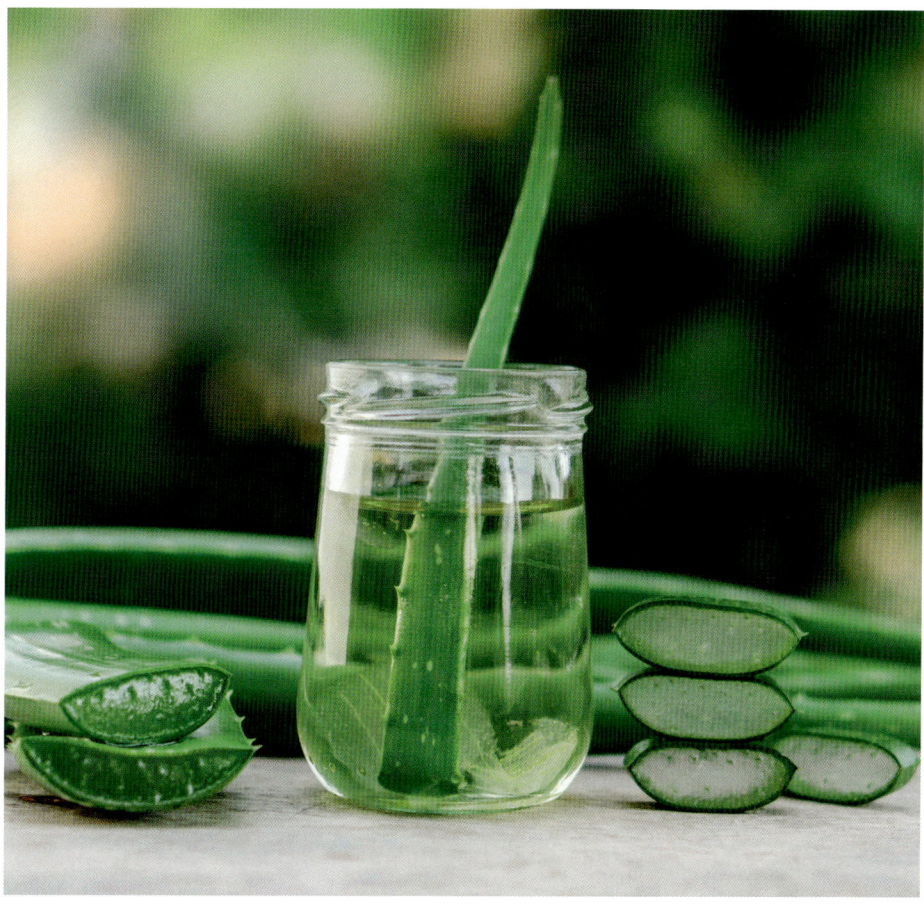

ALOE VERA,
ALOE
BARDADENSIS

know it is spongy and full of fluid, which points to its indications. Similarly, as a flower essence, the Flower Essence Society recommends aloe for "burned out or workaholic syndrome."[16]

Each plant suggests qualities that can be a metaphor for how the plant heals. Likewise, the actual names of plants can offer clues to their healing properties (for example, self-heal is a plant used to assist the body in healing itself after a surgery or accident). Herbal preparations can be consumed orally, in the form of tinctures, teas, infusions, decoctions, powders, and whole foods; or topically, as salves, balms, creams, oils, poultices, smoke, and more. Herbal medicine is generally considered a much safer alternative to allopathic medicine (mainstream medicine that utilizes pharmaceuticals to suppress symptoms), with far fewer side effects and much less toxicity. Also, in contrast to many Western approaches, herbalism works to address the underlying cause of an illness, not merely alleviating its symptoms. It focuses on prevention and awareness. Herbal medicines can be responsibly grown or ethically foraged or wildcrafted—making it a very inexpensive modality.

Everything on the Earth has a purpose, every disease an herb to cure it, and every person a mission. This is the Indian theory of existence.

MOURNING DOVE,
Native American author of *Cogewea*

How Nature Heals

There was no question in the old days that nature was alive and that all life was interconnected. This was the accepted understanding in the West up until the scientific revolution in the fifteenth century. At this turning point, the plant kingdom became a separate domain of life, inanimate and unconscious. Seeing nature as containing a life or vital force became criminal, as divinity was separate from the natural world. And anyone claiming to work with nature or plants without adhering to emerging mechanistic principles was condemned. Our dominant culture is still largely connected to that mindset. So here, too, we are asked to go back and remember a different relationship in order to heal our relationship with nature.

Author Stephen Buhner discusses the profundity of connecting with nature and the plant kingdom, stating that the loss of this connection is the root of many modern maladies. With our increased reliance on technology and pharmaceuticals, we are more vulnerable than ever to separation from our hearts, from nature, and from Spirit. So herbal medicine need not be a physical application, but a journey with a plant or a walk among the trees. Stephen Buhner writes, "As you develop your sensitivity, you can feel the plant begin to move toward you, respond to you, engage with you, entrain with your heart. You can tell, when you pay close attention, the moment when the two of you have established rapport."[17]

CASE STUDY | How Nature Heals

When I met Nina, I felt that her problems were, in large part, being exacerbated by living in New York City, and were mostly situational. She had become very sensitive to her surroundings (she was and remains highly empathic and psychic) and felt depressed in the city, reiterating in our sessions that "the city is sucking the soul out of me." She and her partner were hoping to move to Vermont in the new year, but there were still some financial and logistical hurdles they would have to overcome first.

One of Nina's soul goals was to cultivate her attunement to the plant kingdom and nurture a deeper connection to nature. We brainstormed ways for her to do this while still living in her apartment in Brooklyn. We visualized what her new home and land would look and feel like. As her move became imminent, I gave her a blend to assist her in adjusting to her new environment: walnut for the transition, angelica to feel supported and safe, and bells of Ireland to open up to the nature kingdom of her new property in Vermont.

At our first meeting after she found the property that she and her partner would later purchase, she cried with happiness telling me of the birch tree that had welcomed her to the land. This new plant friend introduced her to the other nature and animal spirits of the property. She felt completely confident and ecstatic about the new world she was moving into. In Nina's case, the lack of actualization she felt was directly related to being disconnected from the Earth. After six months in the country, most of her previous symptoms of exhaustion and anxiety were completely gone.

Not everyone has the opportunity to move out of a challenging environment, and Nina fully acknowledged the privilege of being able to leave the city. Sometimes we must remain in a place even when it feels difficult or not in alignment—there will always be tradeoffs. Luckily, there are other ways to connect with nature even if you live in an urban area, and obviously, flower essences can facilitate this.

A contemporary finding on how nature heals is shown by the study of positive and negative ions in our environments. Positive ions are molecules that have been stripped of an electron (usually in the form of carbon dioxide) and are associated with air pollution. Positive ions have deleterious effects on our systems, causing symptoms such as fatigue, tension, anxiety, depression, allergies, asthma, and endocrine and immunological disorders. They are associated with bacterial and viral infections and many inflammatory conditions, like heart disease and autoimmune disorders. They can be found in places with air conditioning, forced-air heat, fluorescent lighting, Wi-Fi, electrical equipment and outlets, and synthetic materials. Negative ions, on the other hand, are molecules with an extra electron. Negative ions are beneficial to our health, enhancing mood, energy levels, concentration, sleep, and our endocrine and immune systems. Negative ions actually have the ability to attach to bacteria and viruses and neutralize their effects. These ions encourage the brain to produce alpha and theta waves, two frequencies that promote deep relaxation and creative insight. They can be found in nature, especially around waterfalls, oceans, mountains, caves, and forests, and after thunderstorms.[18]

In Japan, *shinrin-yoku*, or forest bathing, further confirms the theory behind the positive effect of negative ions. In part from the dispersal of volatile oils in woodland trees, it has been found that forest bathing reestablishes the yin-yang balance of the parasympathetic and sympathetic nervous systems; decreases blood glucose levels significantly; lowers cortisol, blood pressure, and stress hormones; and has a balancing effect on the endocrine system.[19]

Studying plants for medicinal use gives us the opportunity to observe the patterns of plants, disease, and health. The healing qualities can be understood as tissue states: warming, cooling, drying, moistening, relaxing, and toning. Additionally, grounding is a particular energetic that I reference frequently in my practice, as I feel there is a great need for this direction of energy healing. Tissue states of the body correlate to those of the mind and "your issues become your tissues." Disease and health states also have energetics, such as a wet cough or a heavy depression. Applying the energetics of a plant to encourage balance within a person's physical and/or emotional state is my personal preference for working with herbal medicine.

There are some basic differences between herbal preparations and flower essences. Herbal preparations are different from flower essences in that they contain physical constituents of plants. Herbal tinctures are extracted with the aid of a solvent like alcohol, glycerin, or apple cider vinegar. They can be eaten as a food, ground up into a powder to be ingested, or cooked into a salve to be applied topically, among other things. An energetic or homeopathic dose of an herbal preparation involves using a very small amount of an herbal medicine with the intention of working vibrationally, because smaller doses actually have the potential to penetrate more deeply into the system. (Less is actually more with homeopathy and flower essences.) Also, the actions of a plant may or may not be the same for both an herbal preparation and a flower essence. For example, white-colored flowers, such as boneset, can indicate a connection to bone health in herbalism; however, as a flower essence, boneset is used to address the fear of aging. However, it is also likely that part of the signature will be present in both methodologies. For example, lavender acts on the central nervous system as an herb and as a flower essence. This can be confusing. I consider flower essences to be herbal preparations that are intended to be used vibrationally and to support the subtle anatomy or psycho-spiritual concerns. It makes sense, then, that perceiving flower essences requires more subtlety and intuition than mere physical interpretation.

Vibrational Medicine

Flower essences are individual essences or blends of essences, sometimes called flower essence tinctures, which are charged with a particular frequency of subtle energy and are a form of vibrational or subtle energetic medicine. Vibrational medicine may be the oldest form of healing on our planet. While it is not imperative to subscribe to a particular theory of our true origins, it is useful to consider what it might have been like to exist in a time and within a civilization of deep harmony. The technology utilized by our ancestors was at one time highly sophisticated, eclipsing our current technological advances but with zero waste or corruption. Their advanced frequency technology was applied to every facet of life: engineering, communication, agriculture, and healing. People were attuned to nature to such a degree because survival was dependent on perceiving all subtle natural patterns.

The level of vibration was the pervading level of consciousness to the ancient ones. Education within the Egyptian mystery schools included both physical and subtle

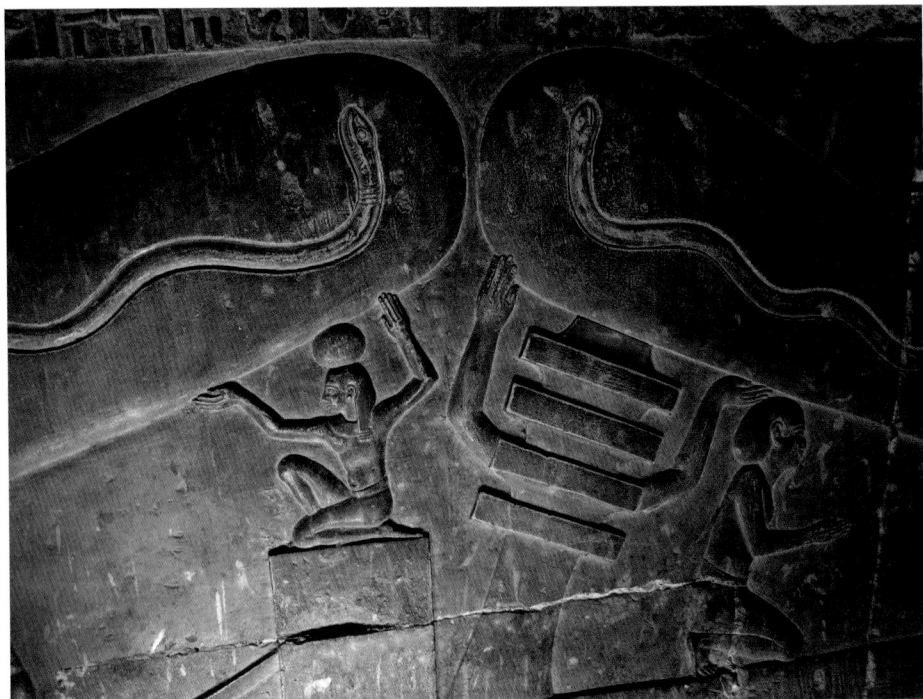

MYSTERIOUS RELIEF DEPICTING LEVITATION. Dendera, Egypt.

training, and students were taught to access information through thought and astral projection. Auric fields, frequencies, subtle energy, the subtle bodies, sound, energetics—these were the levels they were working on. Instruments creating harmonic resonance, sacred geometry, crystals, metals, and plants—these were their therapeutic tools. They also thought of the human self as a divine energy center, and dance and song were vital parts of healing. Much of this level of healing can be found in the sacred practices of indigenous people worldwide.

All knowledge from this era is not lost, but it is a little too abstract for even some in the alternative healing community to accept it as true. While modern science validates many of the laws of vibrational medicine, it is still currently on the periphery of what we perceive as possible and real. In his revolutionary book *Energy Medicine: The Scientific Basis*, James L. Oschman makes the case for the potency of energy medicine. He also asserts that the knowledge of energy medicine is something that is already ingrained somewhere in our consciousness, but that we need to remember it in order to access and apply it.[20]

It's a good idea for us to develop a working knowledge of vibrational medicine because it will continue to proliferate as a powerful branch of healing, and because the Earth and her inhabitants need it. Like the moon consciousness inside of us, vibrational language is something many already grasp, and it is associated with many Eastern, esoteric, mystical, and indigenous teachings. Many of us with clairvoyant/clairaudient/clairsentient abilities already conceptualize from a vibrational or energetic level, feeling thought forms or seeing the subtle bodies or parts of the auric field. Synesthesia, a phenomenon that is becoming increasingly studied, is the blending of experiencing stimuli with the five senses, such as hearing color or feeling numbers. I wonder if synesthesia isn't an enhanced ability to synthesize energy. The vibrational or energetic level is profoundly connected to consciousness. Here, I attempt to summarize the basics. This synopsis is derived from my own experience, plus multiple sources, including the work of Steiner, Oschman, and Richard Gerber, author of *Vibrational Medicine*.[21]

Any modality that intentionally engages the subtle bodies is working at the vibrational level. Some other forms of vibrational or subtle energetic medicine include acupuncture, Reiki, polarity therapy, core energetic therapy, bioresonance therapy, and homeopathy. Additionally, many holistic healing models include aspects of vibrational medicine, such as traditional Chinese medicine (qi), Ayurveda (prana), and craniosacral therapy (breath of life).

Useful Facts about Vibrational Medicine

Everything has a vibration (frequency or resonance), even things that are seemingly inert. This includes thoughts, beliefs, emotions, memories, and geographical places.

Energy cannot be created or destroyed, only moved, accessed, released, or transformed.

All matter can be understood as frozen light. Humans are literally light bodies.

The law of resonance, closely connected with the law of attraction, is the universal law, which determines what you're attracting into your life based on the resonance or frequency/vibration of the energy that you are projecting.

Projected energy can only harmonize with energies that resonate at a similar vibrational frequency, which determines and creates physical results.

Vibration can create matter; for example, cymatics or water structures.

Disease equals lower vibration; health equals higher vibration.

The higher vibrational domain is associated with love; the lower domain is associated with fear, which is associated with trauma. Health and illness are organized around these two polarities, respectively.

Vibrational medicine travels via the crystalline network and the subtle energetic network of the subtle bodies. An example of these channels are the meridians accessed in acupuncture. The chakra system and lesser nadis are another example of the centers and pathways of the subtle bodies.

Energy tends to follow the pathway of least resistance. Water, which makes up the greater part of the human body, is known to be a good conductor of both electrical and subtle energies.

One doesn't need to believe in vibrational medicine for it to work; resonance is a law of nature and a natural phenomenon.

Here's one element of vibrational medicine that seems to be especially difficult for some people to swallow, likely because of its metaphysicality. Vibrational medicine acknowledges the impact of other energetics on the healing process, many of which extend outside of the physical, 3-D domain. Factors that can affect the efficacy of vibrational medicine include:

- the ego
- the subconscious
- the unconscious
- thought forms—one's own and other people's
- natural law

- karma
- our ancestors and ancestral trauma
- prayer and intention
- divine grace

Within the vibrational system, the physical body sits at the center of the subtle bodies: first etheric, then astral/emotional, mental, and finally the causal body, also sometimes referred to as the higher self. They all lie on top of one another, more or less, and are connected via energetic channels, the crystalline network, the chakra systems, and nadis. All subtle bodies are connected to the chakras; however, the etheric has the most active connection.[22] A person's aura is made up of these subtle bodies—this is our subtle anatomy. The self is also connected to a person's guides in the angelic and the celestial realms. Intergenerational trauma comes in with the individual at birth and may imprint on any layer of the self.

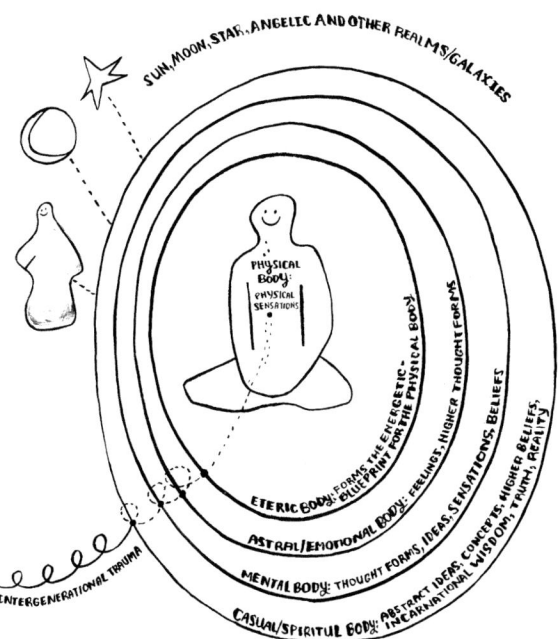

EXERCISE | Subtle Bodies

Let's try to connect with your subtle bodies. Sit comfortably somewhere quiet and close your eyes or set your gaze low. Take some deep breaths into your belly and try and relax. Begin to sense into your physical and subtle bodies. Notice how it feels inside yourself and then outside yourself, in the field around you. Now open your eyes and draw anything that arose during your time tuning in. You might use a corresponding color that feels right for each subtle body. If you're not sure, just go with your intuition. Spend a few minutes with each of your subtle layers. Can you get a sense of them? List some characteristics of each one. What is stored in each layer? What does that look like?

*Beauty is the imprint of the cosmos,
with the help of the etheric body, on a physical, earthly being.*

RUDOLF STEINER

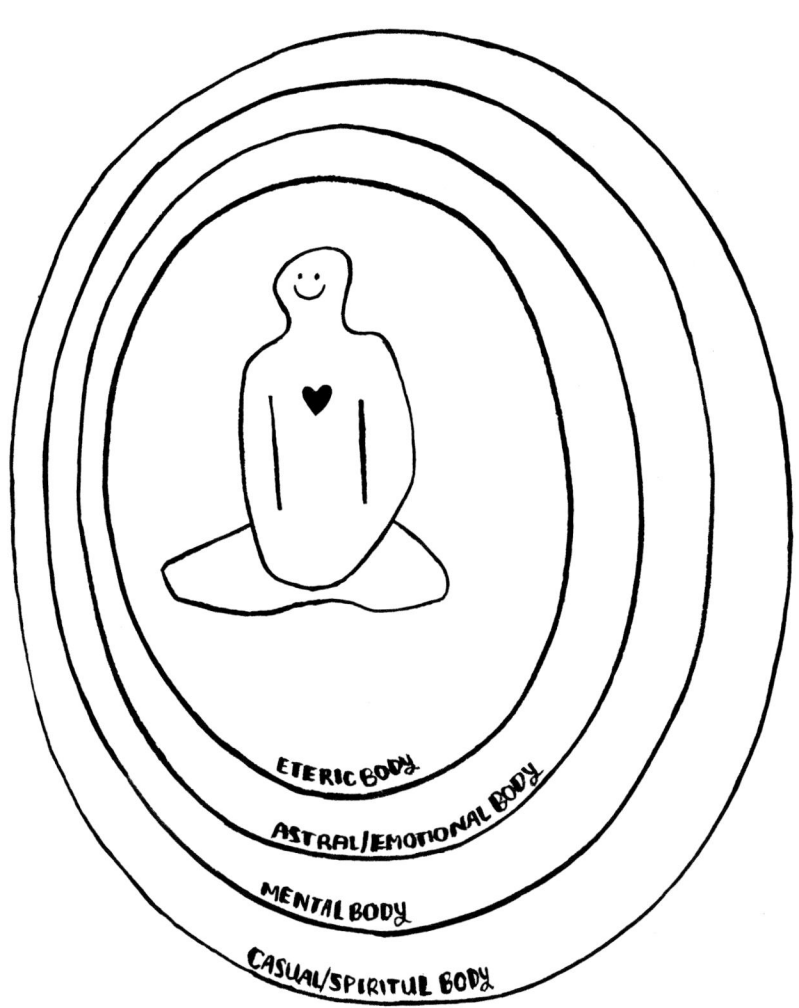

VIBRATIONAL VOCABULARY

Astral/emotional body: Composed of astral matter, this is a subtle substance of even higher energetic frequencies than etheric matter. The emotional body is part of the chakra system. It governs desires and fears and is connected to the physical body via the etheric body. It can be engaged when a person is asleep, and it is associated with near-death experiences, out-of-body experiences, and astral projection. Astral subtle matter is highly magnetic, attracting and repelling energy.

Causal or spiritual body: This exists in the frequency range beyond the mental body; it stores all the lifetime experiences acquired in the reincarnation system.

Crystalline network: Biocrystalline structures that form a network within the body, made up of interstitial fluid, cell salts, fatty tissues, lymph tissue, red and white blood cells, and the pineal gland. These physical structures interact with the subtle bodies to orchestrate the distribution of vibrational medicines.

Einsteinian paradigm: Human beings are networks of complex energy fields that interface with physical/cellular systems; contrasts with the Newtonian system. Electrons can behave as both waves and particles.

Energetic network: This represents the physical/cellular framework, and is nourished by the subtle energetic systems, which coordinate the life force within the body.

Etheric body: This forms the blueprint for the physical body's health and/or illness. In death, this body separates from the person and returns as free energy to the Universe. Etheric subtle energy exists at a higher octave (frequency) than the physical body. Etheric matter is referred to in Eastern esoteric literature as "subtle matter," which is less dense than physical matter; that is, of a higher frequency.

Frequency: The higher the frequency of matter, the less dense or more subtle the matter is. Frequency is a measurement of sound, typically calculated by the number of sound vibrations per second. Frequency is divided into octaves. All matter has frequency. Matter of different frequencies can coexist in the same space.

Holographic principle: Every piece contains the whole and can create an energy interference pattern; every cell within the human body contains the information to create an entire duplicate body: "As above, so below. As within, so without."

Mental body: This exists in the frequency range beyond the astral body.

Magnetism: All electrical fields and subtle matter contain magnetic fields; all magnetic fields generate electrical fields. Every material is influenced by some level of magnetic field.

Negative space/time: All subtle bodies operate in this domain; past, present, and future exist simultaneously.

Physical body: The physical body depends on the etheric body for survival.

Resonance: Tuned oscillators will only accept energy in a narrow frequency band.

Subtle: Referring to energy, matter, and the bodies at a finer resonance than the physical, denser, level.

Subtle bodies: Those psycho-spiritual planes of the self, which exist outside of the physical body, including the etheric, astral, mental, and causal. They are distinct layers but are connected via energetic pathways.

Subtle matter: Denser subtle energy, this can exist in all the subtle bodies. Astral subtle matter is especially magnetic.

Thought forms: Conscious or unconscious thoughts existing in the astral and mental body, these may have emotional intensity, making them denser.

Potentials for Quantum Healing

One of the most exciting components of vibrational medicine is the enhanced potential for healing, beyond what we currently conceive as possible. For millennia, many healers and mystics have tapped into the reality that healing one's field creates quantum healing in others and in the world. This phenomenon is magnified when combined with other tools of resonance. The theory of dissipative structures was developed by Nobel Prize winner Ilya Prigogine, and has some very interesting implications for science such that the critical mass needed for a major change can be accomplished by relatively small shifts in energy.[23] Malcolm Gladwell has a similar idea called the tipping point. Individually and collectively, healing crises provide the impetus for these threshold moments of change.[24]

Vibrational medicine points to the reality that a group of energies or individuals doesn't merely equal the sum of its parts, but that their convergence is exponential. This would mean that when two people come together and hold a particular intention, the energy of that intention produces dramatically more energy than if their individual energies were simply added together. Think of the implications this has for global healing and the anti-oppression, social healing, and justice movements. We hold so much power when we come together and use our energy intentionally. This also gives new meaning to the personal and spiritual work so many are doing. I honor all beings, especially those who have come into their lifetimes with tremendous adversity and suffering. Theirs is the karma of transmuting much darkness into light. They and we do not engage in this process alone. All that is done to heal one's own field impacts the collective and the Earth.

Vibrational Medicine and the Moon

Traditionally, the physical and mental bodies were represented by the sun, and the etheric and astral bodies by the moon. It's no surprise that the domains of the sun have been glorified in medicine, and those of the moon discredited, even labeled evil. This unique, intimate relationship with the etheric and astral bodies applies moon consciousness on another level when utilizing vibrational remedies. Vibrational medicine and the moon share many similarities. They involve many of the more divine feminine characteristics (such as gentleness, receptivity, and engaging one's intuition). The life force of the moon influences plants' growth patterns and life cycles, on both physical and subtle levels. Everything that has been hidden, denied, and vilified represents a huge well of untapped healing potential. Vibrational medicine leaves space for the reality that "healing involves a spectrum of phenomena."[25] Vibrational medicine holds a special role in the realms of moon consciousness, as allowance is made for the transpersonal, the unknowns, and the harmonic technology of the ancients.

Astrologer and herbalist Lata Chettri-Kennedy says this of working with the moon:

I always take into account the planetary alignments before making any herbal medicines or elixirs, and it doesn't have to be that complicated. A lot of the causes of our maladies are a lack of connection with nature and with the elements. One doesn't have to know about astrological omens or any of the planetary aspects to include an awareness of the elements into their own healing. The moon lends herself so easily into the awareness of everyone. We can, wherever we may live, be it in rural or urban areas, follow the cycles of the moon.

We are 70 percent water. We all know the moon is responsible for the ebb and flow of the tides. She affects us constantly whether we know it or not. Working consciously with the moon is the easiest way to connect with your shadow/intuitive side. Simply by witnessing and acknowledging the moon we are placing our intuition in the forefront of our senses where we are more likely to incorporate it in our daily life. We need not live in the woods to be connected to this magical intuitive energy that guides us all. All we have to do is look up.[26]

A huge advantage in working with vibrational medicine is the implicit understanding of how thought influences outcome. Working intentionally is discussed throughout this book, and it is here that vibrational medicine and plant medicine really shine. As more people are awakening to the reality of how vibration leads to creation, where you decide to place your energy becomes an integral part of your work. This goes for individual growth as well as anything physical you create (art, medicine, food, and so on). The more discerning you are with your energy (in what you choose to think about, in what behaviors you decide to engage in, in what stories you keep retelling), the more energy you are giving to possible outcomes.

The moon and vibrational medicine represent those parts of the whole that have been waiting in the wings for the right time in our evolution to be of service again to the mainstream. When we open up healing to include the spiritual sphere, we allow for so much more of the human experience that affects our health. Because all these factors can be understood and worked with on an energetic level, you gain the opportunity to work with the energetics of the plants, the factors underlying health and disease, and much cosmic energy. It's not limited by time and space, by hierarchy, or by validity based solely on physical outcomes. It's an incredibly sophisticated and intuitive way to work. Most of us have been steeped in the mechanistic polarity of health, but coming into cosmic balance is possible when we move toward engaging the subtle and vibrational levels.

Cultural Appropriation and Colonization Within Western Herbalism and Flower Essence Therapy

Working with plant medicine requires us to take responsibility for knowing where the wisdom we are accessing in order to heal comes from, and offer credit and gratitude when appropriate. It is a great disservice to the plants and the people who preserved sacred plant intelligence when we overlook the history and ethnobotany of a plant or practice. Just as we always ask permission to work with a plant, we, too, must ask permission to access the information from other sources.

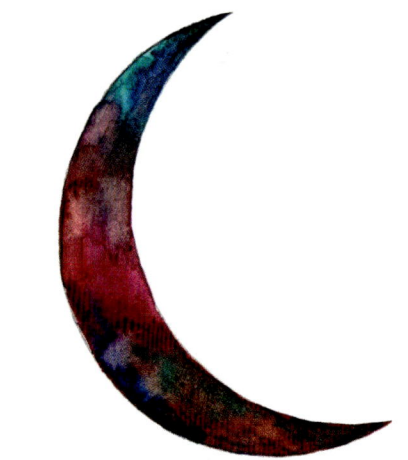

Herbalism and holistic/alternative healing are connected to much ancient and indigenous wisdom, so it generally draws people who are open to nondominant paradigms of healing, but it doesn't preclude that these milieus be free of discrimination. A lot of time herbalism spaces can be just as excluding and oppressive as mainstream spaces. Health care—both Western and natural—is a right, not a privilege, but sadly that is not the case in the US. The issues of oppression and appropriation continue to be a problem that must be addressed if we want to make plant and vibrational medicine and flower essences more accessible and therapeutic for all people, especially marginalized groups. True liberation occurs when we heal together.

Historically, Western herbalism has proliferated within a context of white supremacy, sexism, gender essentialism, classism, and ableism. It has had a pretty fraught relationship with colonization and the appropriation of indigenous medicine and spiritual practices. A lot of European folk traditions were handed down from the Greek humoral tradition, but much of that wisdom came from Egypt and Africa, which is hardly ever mentioned. In addition to mass genocide and slavery, North American and European colonizers took tremendous advantage of traditional Native Americans, European, and African healing practices, co-opting them as their own. Besides stealing plant medicine and practices from black slaves in the antebellum South, white physicians also separated black herbal traditions into what was valid for their use, and branded anything connected to spirit and superstition as invalid and even evil.[27] In America, eclectic medicine evolved out of the plant practices of Native Americans. Many herbal practices were based on oral traditions, are cultural property of distinct groups, and were not necessarily meant to be shared with the mainstream; however, the practices were wrongfully taken and widely assimilated in many cases. This is not to say that there are European and American herbalists who have sought to adopt and share indigenous herbal medicine respectfully and honestly, but the problem generally remains widespread and ongoing.

Decolonizing is about reclaiming what was taken and honoring what we still have.
TINA CURIEL ALLEN

Colonization occurs when a dominant system assumes power and exploits the people and land it takes ownership of. In order to decolonize herbalism and flower essences, we must assess how our ideologies, frameworks, and practices may be doing harm to certain groups and the Earth. We must also challenge the superiority and privilege Western herbalism perpetuates relative to other traditions, as well as honor and support the restoration of indigenous wisdom. Decolonizing our roots is the process of becoming curious about our own heritage and connecting with our own physical ancestry for support. For example, recently I began studying some of the winter solstice folk traditions of the British Isles where some of my people are from.

Cultural appropriation continues when we steal or borrow from a culture without asking for permission, giving credit, or offering compensation—all for our own personal gain. This includes herbal and spiritual indications and practices, such as referencing a native plant or borrowing a ritual without offering credit to how that medicine was used ancestrally. Cultural capital is a valuable commodity in the modern alternative healing landscape. Being particularly sensitive in this way requires diligence as the line between supporting other cultures and appropriating from them can be blurry. Can we bring more mindfulness to herbal practices that originate in cultures different from our own? Can we invest the time and energy into understanding exactly how we've engaged in colonization—of physical, intellectual, and spiritual property? For instance, as a white settler who sometimes wildcrafts medicine in Vermont, in addition to asking the plants for permission before harvesting them (and confirming they are not on the endangered list), I have asked permission of the ancestors and researched the history and people of the land where I'm working.

I used to get so upset when I was just setting out studying shamanism and plant spirit medicine, because of the ways people would respond to me. It took me awhile to recognize my rage was actually in response to the incredible racism and cultural insensitivity that occurs when people make assumptions about indigenous plant medicine. I, too, have a relationship with these plants and practices, and I feel very protective of them.

Indigenous and native medicine people were and are essential to the well-being of their communities and ecosystems. Indigenous practices are not primitive, savage, or unsophisticated. They are simply not of the dominant culture. Under the rule of colonization, many healers were/are deemed primitive and even possessed because of the negative association with magic and witchcraft, despite the efficacy and positive impact these healers have on their communities. In many parts of the world, such as in Africa, practicing traditional medicine under colonial law was punishable by death. With the spread of Christianity, schools of plants were renamed Christian names lest they retain their pagan, and thus sinful, names. The church and secularization were also responsible for the widespread persecution and murder of women throughout Europe and the Americas from the thirteenth through the nineteenth centuries, for folk-healing practices that had always been in use. Some estimates for the number of people executed by the church in Europe during that time are as high as millions, and their persecution still contributes to the negative stigmatization of wise-women healers in the West.[28]

These are but a few examples that are not meant to disparage or discourage, but intended to elucidate how deeply this trauma is embedded in the collective. White settlers now live on stolen land, we borrow stolen practices, and we exploit stolen indigenous wisdom, and most people are completely oblivious to this. We actually celebrate holidays (holy days) that were markers of mass genocide (for example, Thanksgiving). This sustained trauma was occurring over hundreds of years and then ignored by the dominant culture; the reparation from this injury is not something we can just fix overnight.

Flower essence therapy was born out of the Western herbal and homeopathic traditions, and is subject to the same level of contextual oppression, and therefore colonization, as Western herbalism. The founders of flower essences are all white, European men of upper-middle-class status. It's difficult to draw the same correlations to the history of vibrational medicine as it's much more diffuse and varied, but it is more amalgamated from culturally and geographically diverse regions and traditions. There is a lack of diversity among the authors of flower essence literature (I include myself in this list) and larger-scale producers. Flower essences are a type of herbal medicine, and there is much overlap between their indications and practices, as knowledge of their healing properties derives from the same origins and theories. Liz Migliorelli of Sister Spinster is an herbalist and flower essence practitioner who has recently opened up the conversation to include topics of decolonizing one's roots and the role of this work in herbal practices.[29]

I advocate for my flower essence teachers here: Claudia Keel, Patricia Kaminski, and David Dalton have all addressed issues of misogyny, race, and colonization within their teaching models. I owe them much for expanding my knowledge around alternative healing models that challenge Western, patriarchal structures in health and wellness as well as economic and environmental ones. All my teachers have supported understanding the historical and ethnobotanical implications of the herbs and flowers with which one is working; however, this work is ongoing, and deeper levels of understanding the embeddedness of oppression are needed in flower essence therapy.

Having studied the Egyptian mysteries and alchemy, I have always shared a connection to the European alchemical tradition, which greatly informed Paracelsus, whose work was foundational for Hahnemann, and later Dr. Bach. Jane and I have had numerous conversations about what it means for white women to be identifying so strongly with a tradition that is different from our own physical ancestry. After all, I had the good fortune of traveling to Egypt twice, which is a privilege many people with actual African heritage do not have. Historically, the alchemical traditions in ancient Egypt, as well as in other parts of the Middle East and Asia, are generally overlooked. The word *alchemy* derives from the Arabic "al-kimiya." The ultimate purpose of alchemy in ancient Egypt was the process of transformation via cultivating a heart of gold. Interestingly, as the tradition was adopted throughout ancient Greece and then Europe in the Middle Ages, the goal of alchemy became to turn base elements into physical gold. What a succinct metaphor for the patriarchal transmutation of spirit into materialism.

Flowers are the part of the plant that evolved to be in relationship with its environment, and they help us to do the same. Again, if we're going to embark on studying any healing modality, let us also be sure to understand how this impacts us and our community collectively. As more layers of oppression are revealed, collective trauma is (re)surfacing, and we need ways to move forward from a place of compassionate action. I also wonder, at the risk of complicating matters, if we need to hold space for multiple definitions and frameworks at this time to define how healing justice can be applied to flower essences.

I have more questions than answers, but maybe that's okay. There are so many questions I don't have answers to—this in itself is such a masculine, patriarchal instinct, to want to "fix" the problem to alleviate the discomfort. I'm not supposed to have the answers to these questions. Now is the time for the dominant culture to step down and listen to the voice of those who have been ignored and silenced. (Please see "Healing Justice Flower Essence Allies" in chapter four [page 180] for some of the resources that have been helpful to me in my reeducation.)

Selection and Application: The Language of Plants

The simplest way to understand how to work with flower essences is to spend some time getting to know the plant kingdom. Plants help us to know them by way of their signature. To the ancients, every plant had a story to share. Because opening communication to the plant realm seems crazy and pointless to contemporary humanity, much of this attunement has been lost.

We learn best as children, a time when we are innately attuned to the magic of the natural world. We haven't yet been conditioned to doubt our intuition. One of my herbalism teachers, Richard Mandelbaum, would frequently remind us of the benefit of learning about plants with "beginner's mind" and to honor the wisdom of not knowing and defining everything.

When I was young, I woke up each day feeling genuine excitement as I looked outside. The tree in our front yard was my friend; it told me things, it offered me protection. I would pick honeysuckle in the woods and place it in jars of water in the sun to make "potions." No one told me to do this, as far as I can remember. I do remember a neighbor, who was about four years older than I was, making fun of me when I explained to her I was doing "magic."

It wasn't until I began to study plant medicine that I remembered all I must have intuitively comprehended about the natural world as a child, on much more subtle levels than as an adult. If you ever have the opportunity to make flower medicine with children, it is a true delight!

As infants, we gain our first experiences through our connections with our caregivers and by crawling on the Earth. We naturally attune to and take in the world around us with all our senses. But as adults in today's culture—where technology is frequently favored—the lack of access to and emphasis on nature disconnects us from the Earth, each other, and our own hearts. We are all connected to the macrocosm, and, in my practice, I've observed that even if someone is doing everything right (consuming the right supplements, following a good diet, maintaining an exercise regimen), if they aren't connecting with nature, some pathology presents as a result. Even if your access to nature is limited, a walk through a park or sitting with a tree can suffice. Attuning to the natural world will assist your flower essence education and will support your overall health.

EXERCISE: Plant Attunement

Pick a plant growing in nature. If you don't have access to something wild, it can be a live plant you have in your home, perhaps. It might be one you've been admiring or are curious about. Sit beside it; ask for permission to connect with its spirit. Spend about five to ten minutes with it in meditation. Ask what it would like to share with you. What do you notice? Any feelings, images, or physical sensations? Write down any impressions that come to you. At first, there will probably be a part of you that is skeptical about this exercise, and that is okay. Just see if you can observe that part. Draw what you see. It doesn't have to look like the plant. It can be anything that visually arises for you: lights, patterns, shapes, colors.

Plant Signature: Engaging the Six Senses

Flowers captivate all our senses, especially our sight and smell, with their beauty and (for some flowers) their fragrance. Some herbalists prefer to stay within the bounds of the five senses when observing the signature of a plant. All my flower essence training has emphasized relying on one's higher heart and intuitive faculties when studying the flowers. I generally trust what's arising in my heart more than my mind, and this is one area where I pay special attention to what my heart says about a flower. Nature communicates with her own language, beyond our rational, linear minds, and plants invite us to be in relationship with them in order to know them. It is possible to cultivate the heart and intuition through this relationship with nature; it's something that is wired into our beings. The more we cultivate this relationship with nature and the flowers, the more it is reflected back into knowing ourselves. The healing is reflexive. Rudolf Steiner felt strongly that the study of plants should include sense perception as well as engaging the imagination and intuition.[30] After you've familiarized yourself with the idea of plant attunement and recorded your findings, spend some time with your other sense perceptions: sight, sound, smell, and taste. (I would recommend utilizing the tasting of a flower only if no other information presents itself, as the flower could be poisonous or endangered. If you're not sure, rely on your other senses.) You do not need to harm the plant in order to know it; and if you must pick a flower, always ask permission first.

We must take into consideration the plant comprehensively: all its parts, where it grows, when and how it blooms, how it was used by the ancients. It is commonly assumed that people in the ancestral environment developed herbal expertise by trial and error and by accident. I reject this assumption and believe that people during that time possessed tremendous perception to discern plants' healing properties. I believe they also learned simply from being highly attuned to their environments and from the animals who also used the plants therapeutically.

There is a tendency for a lot of Western-indoctrinated folks to want to apply a simple system to define all plants' healing properties according to their signatures. For instance, red flowers can hold a connection to the root chakra but also to the heart. Or a bitter-tasting plant or flower such as dandelion may point to its use for supporting the liver and its connection to the third or solar plexus chakra; but as a flower essence, it's generally applied for physical and emotional tension. There are no hard and fast rules for these categorizations, and there are always exceptions. The most important thing to remember in engaging your six senses is to try and trust your own personal experience!

Shapes

The topic of shape as it pertains to a flower's healing qualities can get quite complex. Flower essences do differentiate from herbs, and sometimes their signatures and indications overlap; however, sometimes they differ. One of the reasons I decided to become an herbalist was to gain a more thorough understanding of how flowers heal, specifically. Personally, I prefer to learn about flowers in their natural environments; however, I don't have abundant access, as I live in the city. I feel this is one area I could be more fluent in, and hopefully one day I will have the opportunity to fully immerse myself in studying flower shapes in a field in Vermont. For now, I must rely on my intuition and heart sense, and the observations of others, more so than if I were in that field in Vermont.

No one has written more comprehensively on the signatures of the Bach plants than Julian Barnard. In his *Bach Flower Remedies: Form and Function*, Barnard explains, with great detail and delight, the gestures, ecology, and the healing properties of the plants used to make the Bach essences.[31] If you are curious to learn more about flower shapes specifically, I highly recommend *Flowers that Heal*, by Patricia and Richard Kaminski, and Julia Graves's *The Language of Plants: A Guide to the Doctrine of Signatures*, which explores this topic in great detail.[32]

The following are some of the shapes (and their possible meanings or expressions) you may encounter:

- Bell- and tube-shaped flowers can mean something is getting pulled up; or could have a deeper action, and things will come up; for example, the snowdrop for the expression of deeply held trauma.
- Thistles are spikes that have a releasing quality, for example, milk thistle for the release of anger.
- Star-shaped flowers, have an uplifting quality, and connect us to the star realm, for example, shooting star for those who don't feel comfortable on Earth.
- Flat-facing flowers, such as in the Asteraceae or daisy family, can show us where fears are held in our third, or solar plexus, chakra; for example, gloriosa daisy "helps a person to choose, align with and persist in all matters of soul growth."[33]
- Trumpet-shaped flowers connect with communication; for example, trumpet flower for heart-centered communication.
- Tree flowers are generally connected to the first chakra; for example, redwood is used for sacred stability and spinal issues.
- Organ-shaped flowers such as uva ursi, which resemble ovaries, connect with the deep void, the feminine, and are used physically to address the ovaries.

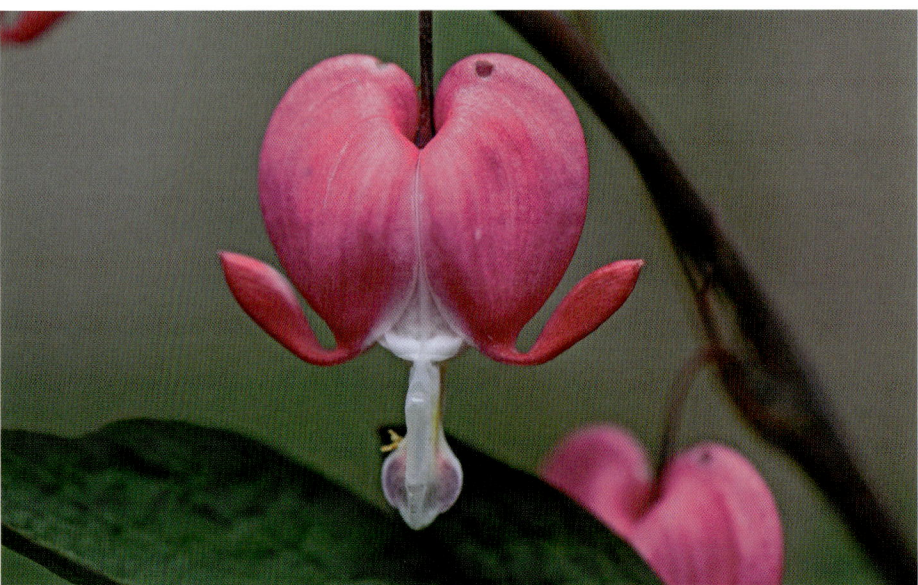

BLEEDING HEART

- Heart-shaped flowers, such as bleeding heart, help us during times of heartbreak and loss.

Other factors to consider:

- What is the flower's orientation? Does the flower open to the sky? Is it pointing toward the Earth? This could indicate a grounding energy (for example, cayenne).
- When does the flower bloom? Flowers in the aster family bloom later in the summer and autumn, which illustrates their usefulness for dealing with aging, death, and loss. David Dalton has a special aster set for support in this area.
- While not technically a flower essence, according to gemmotherapy (a branch of herbalism that utilizes the buds of trees and plants), the energetic potential of the future plant can be harnessed into the medicine, and the use of young plant tissues actually has its own unique therapeutic indications. This is another example of how the energetics of a particular *time* in the plant's developmental stage plays a role in its healing signature.[34]

As we look more deeply at understanding plant signatures, we can see patterns emerge between form and the numbers of petals, and the way the flowers function. Geometry is a mathematical system that serves as a language to understand cosmic balance and divine order. Within the concept of sacred geometry are the ideas of oneness, twoness, threeness, and so on. Sacred geometry recognizes the divinity in the natural shapes of our cosmos. As you will soon discover, plants rarely fit neatly into binary thinking. (In chapter four, Jennifer Patterson of Corpus Ritual will show us how poisonous plants also have healing qualities.) We will build on the relationship between sacred geometry, plant signature, and the flower of life in the next chapter.

The Elements and Elementals

Just as all living things possess a particular vibration, so do they have elemental characteristics. The elements are indicators of the form and function of a plant—they reveal a good deal about the plant's energetic signature. The elementals are the spirits of the elements. In some traditions, such as traditional Chinese medicine, there are five elements: earth, fire, water, metal, and wood. Vedic astrology, too, utilizes the elements in interpreting one's natal chart. I work within the four-element

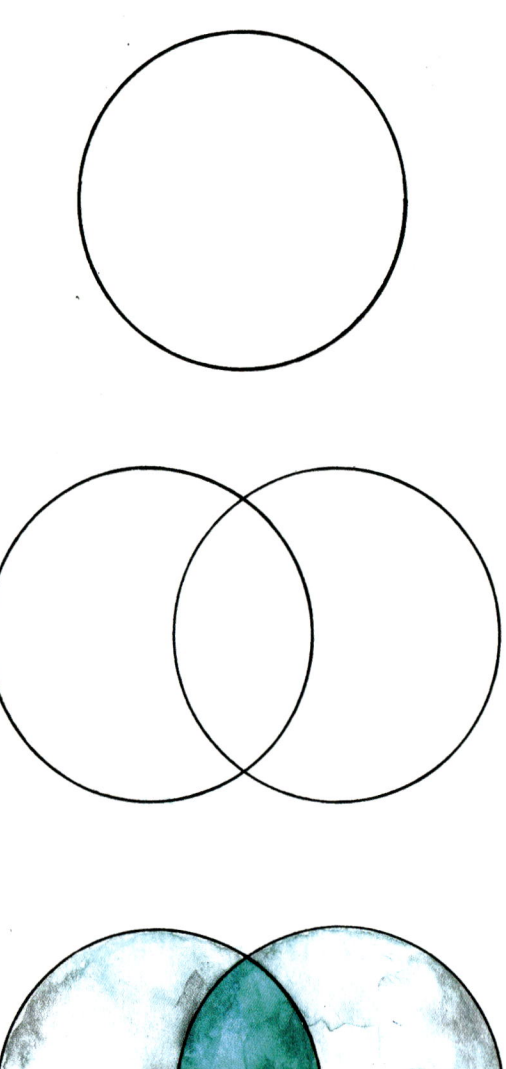

ONENESS
(unity consciousness—
form is the circle)

TWONESS
(the circle divides
and becomes two—
opposition, polarity—
two parts in
relationship to
one another)

THE VESICA
PISCIS is the
shape that two circles
overlapping make—
birth portal,
vertical/horizontal
(eye), how the flower
of life is formed

conceptualization of earth, air, fire, and water. Color, too, is a living aspect of the plant signature. Working with the elements and elementals gives us the ability to see where we can invite more balance into our lives.

The elements can further be divided into feminine and masculine. According to Julia Graves, yin (feminine) and yang (masculine) "are important in the context of the elemental signature, since they represent the primary elemental dyad. Yin and yang are the first polarization that evolves from the all-one."[35] In gaining greater insight into the plants and ourselves, it is possible to ascertain knowledge by applying the wisdom of the elements. The elements are living energies that possess their own consciousness. If you feel a strong connection to the elements, please refer to a more complete list of how the elements speak through their doctrine of signature in Graves's book, *The Language of Plants*.

Selecting Essences

Flower essences can be purchased from a quality producer (such as those mentioned in the Appendix, page 183), or you can make your own. Here, I will discuss how to select and apply ready-made flower essence remedies. How to produce your own flower essences will be discussed in "Formulation: How to Make Your Own Medicine" (page 98).

When you're starting out with flower essences, it can be overwhelming—so many producers and so many essences! I like to encourage people to remember that it's your relationship with the plant that is the most important thing in selection. Your relationship with the remedy is the co-creation with that plant. The more you work with flowers, the more you will be able to feel and trust this part of the process.

The following are some ways to begin exploring flower essences:

- Depending on what issue(s) you'd like to address, begin by taking one to three essences that resonate with you. Many producers offer sets of remedies that have a particular focus. You may want to purchase a set to experiment with, such as the FES's Range of Light, Delta Gardens' Protection Set, Alaskan Essences, or the Bach Essences (see the Appendix for more information).

- Consider flower essences that invite presence, relaxation, protection, and grounding.

- If you want to study the essences more carefully, consider making flash cards or purchasing the flower cards (Alaskan Essences, FES, and Bach make sets).

- If you're curious to learn more about how a plant might connect with your ancestry, consider doing some research on how it was used historically.
- Perhaps there's a flower you're curious about, or have seen in nature. Ask this plant if it would like to work with you.

Here are five basic ways to select a flower essence:

- Intuitively: A flower essence might come to you by way of revealing itself in nature, or appearing in a dream.
- By dowsing: Using a tool of resonance, such as a pendulum, to test for essences.
- Through muscle testing: A simple way to muscle test is to make a ring with the index finger and thumb of your nondominant hand. If you would like to test for a yes for an essence, say the name of the plant and flick the circle with your dominant hand. If the circle holds, that's a yes. If it breaks open, that is a no.
- By consulting reference literature: Books, repertories, or flower affirmation cards.
- Through blind testing: By drawing a card or randomly selecting an essence from a set. This method works well with children.

Any of these methods can be integrated into your ritual. Before making remedies for other people, it's a good idea to spend some time with the flower essences yourself. The flowers will have much to share with you. Also, the more experience you have with the essences yourself, the better you will understand how the essences will work for others.

Intention

Your intention is the reason you feel called to make your medicine. It is the core issue, or situation, you want to address. It is the mission of your medicine. Especially when starting out, it's helpful to consider how to *ground, protect,* and *feel safe*—domains of the first three chakras. These states support presence, a relaxation within the system, and allow a person to drop into new awareness. My intentions are usually focused around balance. For instance, if a client is suffering from shock, I definitely want to help them ground, stay in their bodies, and feel safe, and also stabilize in a way that they can move through the situation. I always include at least one or two essences in my blends for grounding, protection, and safety, and have found that being mindful of these energetics creates a well-balanced formula. Great healing is available to us with the flower essences in the beginning, but it is necessary to understand that there is a progression in the direction of healing that should be respected. I try and keep the intention simple and elegant—too many objectives for one remedy tend to muddle the medicine. If you're unsure about the clarity of your intention, you can always test for it and refine as needed. The perfect condition for setting intentions is when your soul goals are in alignment with what the Universe wants for you (or for someone else). And remember, with subtle medicine, more doesn't equal better.

Setting an intention doesn't mean you control the outcome of the remedy. On the contrary, letting go of a desired outcome frees up more energy for the medicine to work its own magic. In clarifying your intention, consider using positive statements, such as "I'd like to invite in more protection," instead of "I don't want to feel unsafe." Because we are working with resonance, we want to work in the flow of energy we would like to attract, and positive attracts positive. Other questions to consider asking yourself: "What would support me/another person in the highest way right now?" "What do I/another person need to feel safe and grounded?" "What energetics could support this person or situation coming into greater balance?" We want everything we offer up to be for our highest good and highest healing.

Formulation

When you become more familiar with working with flower essences, you may begin to formulate blends of flower essences, known as a tincture or formula. I highly recommend you invest in some kind of formal training with a professional to gain a more comprehensive skill set on this topic as there are limits to being self-taught. The goal of a formula is to combine the energetics and properties of several flowers to match the intention for the remedy. Formulation is a lengthy topic, and I will offer the basics for you to get started.

In my herbalism training, I was taught that when you formulate effectively, there is a potentiating synergy, meaning the individual plants work together to create a particularly potent medicine. (The idea that a medicine's potential can be greater than the sum of its parts connects back to Prigogine's theory on dissipative structures.) In my opinion, it is the thoughtfulness that goes into the intention of the remedy that greatly contributes to this effect.

When formulating, we want to match the remedy to the person *as well as* the pattern of disharmony. Whatever is imbalanced should, of course, be a consideration, but to merely apply a flower essence to address a symptom is a sheerly palliative approach, and we're interested in deeper integration than that. In an herbal formula, one would want to assess contraindications, age, weight, short- and long-term effects, financial/accessibility considerations, and comorbid conditions. Flower essences make formulating simpler in a physical sense, as these factors are less of an issue.

Here is my basic formula for creating a flower essence tincture of three flower essences. It is adapted from my teacher Claudia Keel's methodology and is something I learned early on in my training. Before I begin, I always sit and ground for a few moments and bring my intention for the remedy into my field. I will say my prayer and ask for guidance with any questions I may have. I always make space for guidance to arise beyond my knowing, and I try to get out of the way to allow the formula to flow through me. I will ask: What is required to bring myself or the situation into balance?

I will select:

1 **primary flower essence**—this is the main flower of the blend.
1 **supporting flower essence**—this should be an essence that supports the main flower essence.
1 **balancing flower essence**—this is an essence that has a balancing effect on the other two essences.

Consider the energetics of the primary and supporting essences. If they are both very upward-moving, perhaps they need to be balanced with something grounding and downward-moving.

Thinking back to "Selecting Essences" (page 89), consider how you feel drawn to your selections. It's okay if you're not sure what the primary, supporting, or balancing flower essence should be; you can always test for it.

How you choose to show up magnetizes what shows up for you.
ANONYMOUS

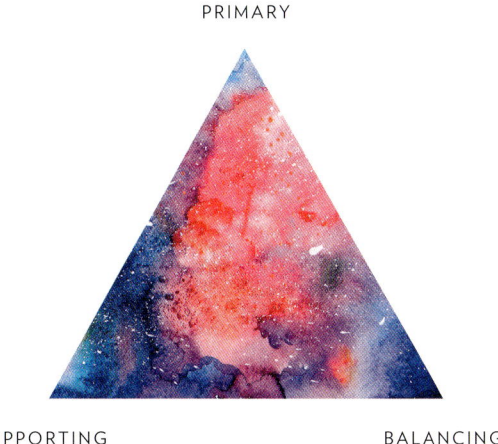

PRIMARY

SUPPORTING　　　　　　　　　BALANCING

The Chakra System at a Glance

In many ancient traditions, the chakras were depicted as flowers. The chakras are a series of energy centers that are located along the central meridian of the body. There are different interpretations of the chakra system, some with up to twelve energy centers, with additional ones outside the body. I work within the framework of the seven-chakra system. Each of the seven chakra points governs a particular area of the body and certain functions. Chakras are like layered orbs, and are very much multidimensional. Their Western corollary is the endocrine system. According to the teachings of David Dalton, it is best to address trauma in the first three chakras first, before moving on to other issues. He feels most of our healing takes place in these areas.[36] The nature of trauma can be multilayered, and the work of healing our core wounding is ongoing—it's not like you heal your issue with your ex-partner in your second chakra one week, and then you're finished. In the cross section of people I see, some common wounds and patterns I observe include: lack of connection to the Earth and one's ancestry (first chakra); sexual trauma, poor boundaries/saying no, creative blocks (second chakra); lack of confidence, inability to trust self, little or confused sense of self (third chakra); inability to give and receive love, inability to be vulnerable, inability to connect with inner wisdom (fourth chakra); unsure or unable to access one's voice, fear of one's power (fifth chakra); intuitive vision blocked (sixth chakra); and disconnected from one's divinity and guides and angels (seventh chakra).

When to Use Flower Essences

One of the best aspects of working with flower remedies is their universal application. Since they are essentially homeopathic, there are no side effects, and they pose no contraindications for children, pregnancy or breastfeeding, or other medications. They are also safe for animals and, in my experience, animals are especially receptive to them. They are appropriate for both acute issues and longer-term use. The Bach Rescue Remedy was produced especially for emergency situations, to create a stabilizing field around a person when significant trauma or shock has occurred. There are essences I have become particularly fond of, ones that I take myself and put in my tinctures for others regularly. Flower essences are a wonderful complement to any kind of therapeutic

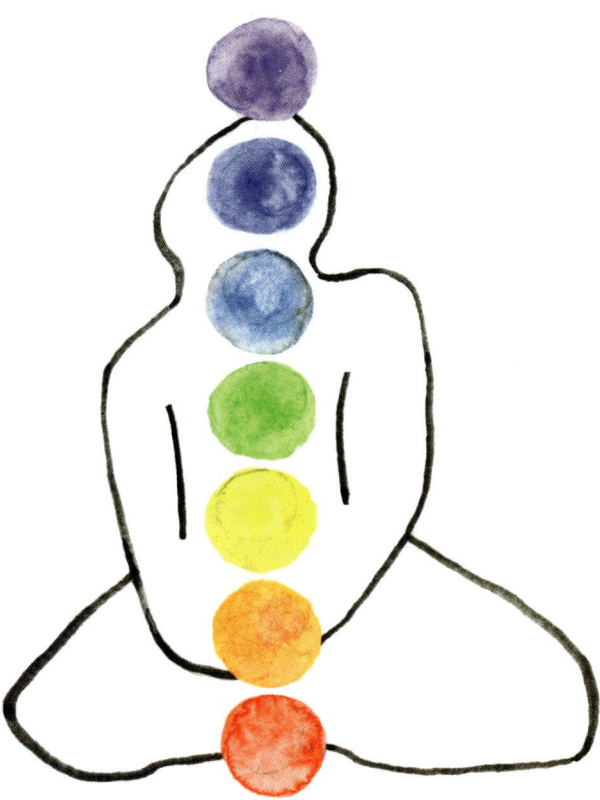

work, as they don't interfere with herbal or medicinal protocols. They can be used as mists to encourage clearing, grounding, protection, or to raise the frequency within a space, such as an office.[37] Dosage will be covered later on, but here I will mention that it is advisable to only work with single or a few remedies at a time.

In acute situations with severe symptoms, such as an accident, emotional or physical trauma, conflict, abandonment, deep grief, terror, severe depression, or suicidality, flower essences are medicines I rely upon and trust. Flowers have become essential to my life's work—those lessons and teachings I'm integrating on a soul level.

I feel it's useful here to elaborate on how the flower essences work their magic in the longer term. The plant spirits seek our highest evolution, and that doesn't always mean getting to skip steps of learning, in grieving, resistance, conflict, or any of the lower vibrational states. It's not that we're supposed to suffer through these times, but the essences aren't going to act as silver bullets, especially if we're meant to integrate a particular experience in our lives. Essences can either assist you in shifting your relationship to the energetics around a particular issue or alleviate it altogether.

I have witnessed dramatic positive shifts in symptoms, interpersonal conflict, life circumstance, and outcome while both personally taking and observing the essences working in others. Sometimes they act in much more sophisticated and mysterious ways than our consciousness can permit us to comprehend. Some essences I always have handy in times of emergency are Bach's Five-Flower Formula, Bloesem's Terra—an Emergency Combination, and Alaskan Essences' Soul Support.

In addition to being applied directly to a healing crisis of a human or animal, flower essences can be applied to other crises holographically. Meaning that, if there is a situation or place that you would like to help, it is possible to hold an intention around that situation or place and make a remedy in service of it. For instance, if you are trying to clear a lot of ancestral trauma in your lineage, you might create a remedy in honor of it. You could work with it in a ritual of some sort, or place it on your altar or in a sacred place in your home. It can be particularly potent to do this work in a group for an environmental crisis. You could gather together, set the intention, and make the medicine together, then offer it up by saying a prayer or singing a song together. Remedies can be dropped ceremoniously into bodies of water and on sacred land, such as a polluted ocean or endangered area, to bless them.

Working with Others: A Word of Caution

When making remedies for others, it is a good idea to assess your level of impartiality. The intention you hold for someone could very likely be different than what would promote their highest good. Generally, it is not advisable to involve yourself in other people's karma. Let me offer an example, because this is crucial to convey. Say you meet with someone who has endured sexual trauma, and they are suffering terribly. Though your intention may be good, in that you want to help them release the trauma, they may not be ready to let go of all the ways in which they have organized their life around the trauma, and dramatically releasing that energy could be destabilizing or dangerous. It is a process, and it may not happen overnight. Always opt for safety and grounding first. Consider all the aspects of the healing process that are part of this journey.

Flower essences work in tandem with the therapeutic process and may not follow a linear path, as our rational minds assume. Working with other people requires great integrity and objectivity. Many unconscious projections can occur in the therapeutic relationship. If it is not possible for you to remain impartial in offering flower essences to someone close to you, spend some more time with the flowers first, and come back to your person later. As a rule, I always ask the soul's permission before formulating for someone.

Ritual

Bringing ritual into your practice is essential for selecting and making flower essences. Allow your ritual to be a unique expression of those practices that feel true and supportive of your intentions. The ritual you choose can be anything that inspires you—a prayer, a mantra, or a song. To be sensitive to cultural appropriation, it's a good idea to understand the history and culture behind your practices.[38] This is also a great opportunity to dive into your own ancestry for inspiration.

Your ritual might include any stones or sacred objects that feel special to you. It might involve lighting a candle or burning some incense. It doesn't have to be fancy or elaborate, but it should be focused and intentional. Working on vibrational levels means we're working with very fine energy. The energies that you bring into your flower essence ritual will be felt and affect the action of the remedy. Bach felt strongly that human beings should have minimal influence on the medicine-making process, so again, keep simplicity in mind.[39]

The timing of when you decide to craft your essence affects its energetic signature. You may choose to work with the energy of a certain time of day or during a particular lunar phase. New moons, full moons, eclipses, and other planetary alignments can be considered based on the energetics you'd like to incorporate. (Additional ritual ideas will be shared in chapter four, "Flower Rituals for Healing and Transformation.")

Application

The classic application of working with flower essences is by taking them orally, under the tongue. There are also so many ways to use them beyond ingesting them. You can add them to oils, lotions, balms, and baths. Mists are a great option for children, pets, and spaces. Used topically, the essences can be felt on a different level. Adding flower essences to a bath can be part of a beautiful care regimen. Gurudas mentions flower essence bathing extensively in his text, *Flower Essences and Vibrational Healing*. Flower essence tinctures can be applied directly onto the skin around particular pulse points, such as the crown, the third eye, or the heart chakra. They can be added to other healing modalities such as craniosacral therapy or acupuncture.[40]

Tinctures usually contain one or three essences at a time, and occasionally five, seven, or nine. We want to honor simplicity, and the ability to connect with each plant spirit. Again, more isn't necessarily better—that's connected to an outdated paradigm. Set aside a few times during the day when you can really concentrate when taking your tincture, such as first thing in the morning or before bed at night. Take three drops of an oral blend three times a day or as needed; if that feels too strong, don't take it before bedtime. Take the tincture for one month, even if in the beginning you notice no changes; the remedy is working on less-discernible levels.

Make time and space to connect with the plant spirits in your blend. Consider taking your tincture in tandem with a meditation practice, a mindful activity, or by simply closing your eyes and taking a few deep breaths each time you take the remedy. You may feel called to integrate your tincture with another healing modality, or any other "way in" you are exploring. If you are working through something really heavy and need more support, consider collaborating with a professional to enhance the integration process.

Formulation: How to Make Your Own Medicine

The way I was taught to make flower essences was handed down from the Bach tradition. Bach also made essences by a boiling method, but I use the sun preparation method. Making your own flower essences can be a magical and joyful experience. It is empowering to make your own medicine, and doing so opens another dimension of consciousness and healing with the plant kingdom. This deeply rewarding ritual is also quite affordable and is available to anyone who can access nature for a few hours.

As with selection, your vibrational signature impacts the quality of the remedy you formulate. This doesn't mean you need to become a monk to make medicine. It does mean that you need to be discerning about your energy; for example, I generally don't make medicine for anyone if I'm having an emotional day. Every tool you use must be clean. The water should be of the highest quality. The idea is to mimic the morning dew.

Here are the tools you will need:

- a thin, clear glass bowl (with no designs)
- one 2-ounce amber bottle for the mother essence
- one 1-ounce amber bottle for the stock essence
- one ½-ounce bottle for the dosage essence
- labels for the bottles
- fresh spring water (from a glass bottle, if possible)
- early morning sunlight (or moonlight or starlight)
- brandy (or apple cider vinegar)
- a clear mind

- for the mother essence: ⅔ flower water and ⅓ brandy solution
- for the stock essence: add 7–10 drops per ounce of ⅔ water and ⅓ brandy solution
- for the dosage essence: add 7–10 drops per ounce of ⅔ water and ⅓ brandy solution

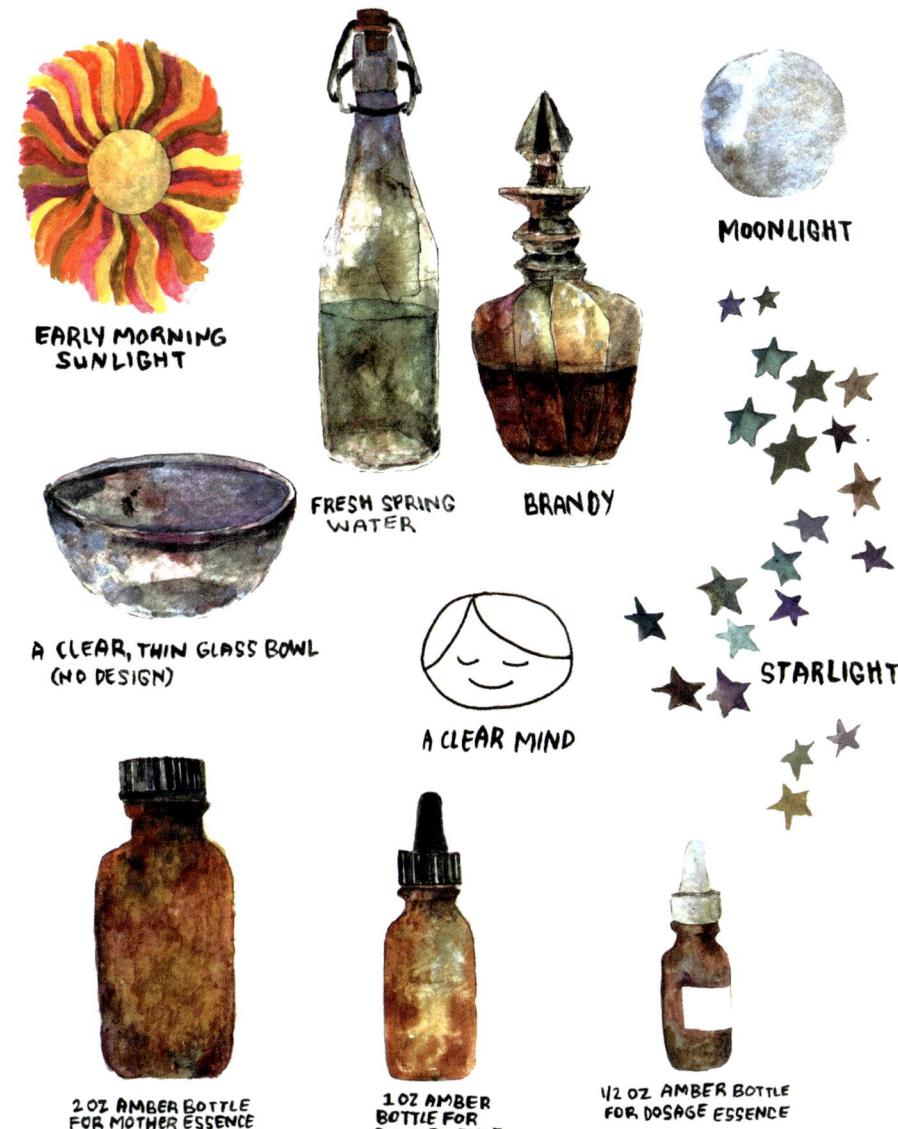

DEW: THE COSMIC WATER SOURCE

The moisture that forms on the Earth's surfaces when atmospheric vapor condenses at night is known as dew. The role of dew in ancient medicine-making points to its unique interface between the physical and subtle realms and its link to the elements. Dew was a particularly magic substance to many ancient cultures, and to physicians and philosophers up through the nineteenth century. Dew was thought to contain all sorts of healing and cosmic properties, such as the abilities to heal skin and dissolve gold. In certain conditions, it appears out of nothing under the cover of darkness, so it was understood as very mysterious and supernatural.

Dew, or celestial waters, was highly regarded in the Western alchemical tradition for its connection to the elements of fire and air (nitre). Nitre was thought to exist at the highest level of physical form, just before the subtle realm, so it is a physical element but very close to being nonphysical. Because water in this form is created from fire and air, it is imbued with a special relationship to transformation. The act of creating medicine from this water, then, blends all the elements (plant being the Earth element) synergistically. Both Hildegard von Bingen and Paracelsus collected dew from flowering plants to be used for treating disease.[41] Dr. Bach believed, as von Bingen and Paracelsus did, that dew collected from plants held the curative imprint from that plant, and so flower essences were a pure and potent form of medicine, and connected to the macrocosm through the four elements.

From the work of Masaro Emoto and some others, we know that water can hold, transmit, and amplify information. This concept is currently highly controversial within the scientific community. However, as our consciousness becomes more attuned to the subtle reality of nature, perhaps our testing measures can validate this more accurately in the future.

Go out into nature in the early morning if you're making a traditional essence. It is wonderful to work early enough that dew is still on the plants. Sunny weather is best, but it's totally acceptable to make essences under other weather conditions. If you're making a moonlight or starlight essence, pick a time of night, but remember that some

MORNING DEW ON LADY'S MANTLE. In the Middle Ages and the Renaissance, women would collect dew from lady's mantle for its skin rejuvenating properties.

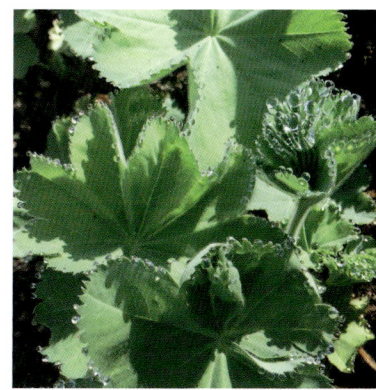

ALCHEMISTS COLLECTING DEW (from the *Mutus Liber*, 1702). Chris Walker Collection/Alamy Stock Photo.

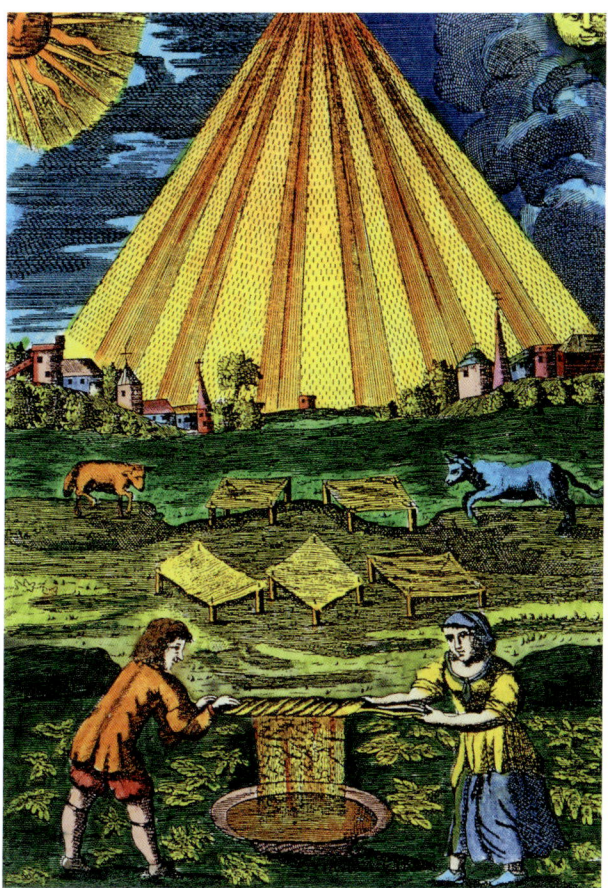

flowers close at night. Select a flower that calls to you. Ask for permission to work with that plant. Consider the land on which you are making your medicine, especially if you are not native to that region. Remember, Western herbalism has a history of taking without asking permission, and we don't want to reinforce harm onto the land and her inhabitants. If permission isn't granted (you receive an intuition of no, or are not sure), it may not be the right time or conditions. Depending on your geographic location, you can use a book such as Newcomb's *Wildflower Guide* or Peterson's *Field Guide to Medicinal Plants and Herbs of Eastern and Central North America* to identify your flower.[42] Avoid using flowers in areas that have been sprayed by pesticides, like urban parks and the sides of roads. It is possible to use flowers from gardens that have been cultivated naturally, although this will alter the vibration of your essence. Making flower essences in urban areas can be challenging. You may need to venture out to find the flowers.

Connect with the spirit of nature, the spirit of your flower, and any other guides you work with, and state your intention. Use your ritual to select which and how many flowers to use, and place them in the glass bowl filled with water. I usually pick flowers in odd numbers. Bach felt the water should be completely covered with flowers, although I don't always follow this rule. Claudia taught me to pick flowers using a leaf, so that no part of you touches the flower. You want to pick only the very top of the plant with the inflorescence (the complete flower head). For endangered or poisonous flowers, just place the bowl of water near the plant instead of harvesting it. If you're not sure which flowers might be poisonous, and the idea of this makes you nervous, simply find another flower. Situate the bowl in the natural environs of the flower.

Now that you have your bowl of water with the flowers in it, sit and be still for two to three hours, whatever length of time you are guided. Heartier flowers may need more time in the sun while more delicate flowers may need less, depending on the outside conditions. It's not necessary to be in perfect meditation for the entire time the flowers are solarizing, but this is a beautiful opportunity to connect with the plant kingdom. I've had pretty psychedelic experiences with guides, plant spirits, faeries, different dimensions, and all kinds of planetary energies during this ceremony. You may wish to journal your impressions at this time. Or you may feel guided to lie down and rest— you may have some interesting dreams!

Whatever you choose to do during this time, try to be mindful and quiet. At the end of the two to three hours, gently take out the flowers and any insects or leaves that are in the water so the water is clear. Use a leaf to take the flowers out of the water and offer them back to the Earth. Take the two-ounce bottle and fill it one-third of the way with the brandy or vinegar. Pour some of the water from the bowl into the bottle with brandy, and offer the rest of the flower water in the bowl back to the Earth. This is your mother essence. The mother can be stored indefinitely; it will not lose its vibration if stored properly.

To make your stock essence, take the one-ounce bottle and fill it a third of the way with brandy or vinegar. Then fill it two-thirds of the way with spring water. Add seven to ten drops of the mother into the stock bottle. The stock essence will last for ten years.

To make your dosage essence, repeat the steps for the stock, except this time only add three to seven drops of the stock to the dosage. Take a half-ounce bottle and fill it one-third of the way with brandy or vinegar, and two-thirds of the way with spring water. Add three to seven drops of the stock into the dosage essence. This essence will stay vibrationally potent for ninety days.

The boiling method of making flower essence is useful for early spring plants that need less sunlight. This method requires the use of an enamel pan on a stove top. In addition to collecting the flowers of a plant, collect leaves and twigs as well. Cut them and allow them to fall directly into the pot. Immediately bring the pot inside and fill with spring water. Use ten parts water to one part plant material. Boil uncovered for half an hour. Remove all plant material with a twig, let cool, and pour through a paper filter into a clean clear bowl. Follow the instructions for the sun method in bottling the mother, then stock, and dosage essences.

Storing Essences

Flower essences are sensitive, and the way you store them affects their potency. Care should be taken to create a calm and quiet place for your essences. They are best kept in your care only. I don't let anyone else handle my remedies.

The following are some basic rules for storing your essences:

- Keep them in a cool place (between 65 and 80 degrees Fahrenheit) that's also dry and dark.
- Keep them away from electromagnetic frequencies (electrical outlets, Wi-Fi routers, cable boxes, or cell phones).
- Keep them out of reach of pets and small children.
- Store them upright.

- Keep them separate from essential oils, or their volatile constituents will penetrate your flower essences.
- Seasonally or yearly, test your essences for potency and discard any that have developed any mold or bacteria, or that feel energetically less active.
- Monthly, seasonally, or yearly, cleanse your essences by whatever means you like: singing bowls, chimes, sage, and the like.

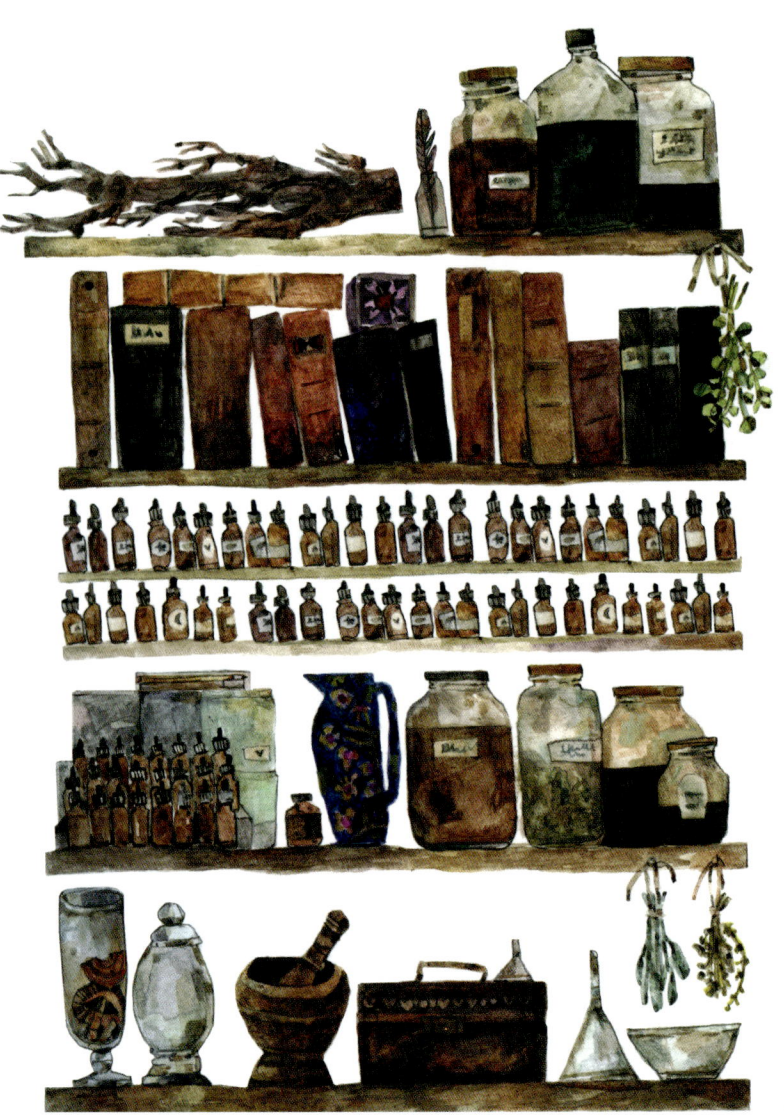

Man's attitude toward nature today is critically important simply because we have now acquired a fateful power to alter and destroy nature. But man is part of nature, and his war against nature is a war against himself.

RACHEL CARSON, Silent Spring

Women Healers Throughout History

Missing from our Western history books are most of the contributions by women-identified healers through the ages. Even more scarce are queer and trans people of color (QTPOC) within the codex of Western medical history. The misogyny of the burgeoning patriarchy from ancient Greece spread throughout Europe, Africa, the Americas, and the rest of the world through colonization by white settlers. The suppression of women healers in Europe and the Americas coincided with the rise of the ruling class, capitalism, and the privatization of medical care, away from folk-healing traditions—traditions that women played a huge role in preserving and advancing. Gender seemed to be less of a construct throughout many parts of the ancient world, as there are significant written reports of intersex and gender-fluid healers. In many cases, those who exhibited androgyny were known as having special healing powers because of their ability to connect with both masculine and feminine energy.

As historical contexts are becoming more inclusive and less Eurocentric, there is more room for the theory around matriarchal-centered civilizations being much more prominent than previously thought. Senegalese anthropologist and historian Cheikh Anta Diop felt that, historically, most of Africa was matriarchal in organization.*[43] Colonizers were tremendously misogynistic, which holds much information for us to ponder as we consider our connection to the feminine and the history of medicine.

The lack of representation of women and WOC healers in the historical literature of medicine is decidedly a Western trait. Not only is much history transmitted orally and through practices and traditions, but the written history is also a very biased account, formulated in large part by, and for, white men. While our participation in medicine and healing traditions has been historically restricted in the West, women

---

* This is not to say that the matriarchal societies dominated the patriarchy, rather, there was "a harmonious dualism."

have long been associated with healing, especially within the domains of life and death—as midwives and compassionate caregivers helping to bring new life and support the soul into the afterlife. Women healers have traditionally addressed the issues and needs of populations that our culture typically shames and would rather ignore. Written accounts are limited, but we do have a record of a talented few. We must honor the oral traditions that are not meant to be shared (by me anyway) with the mainstream. There is a protection in keeping knowledge hidden from the masses. This wisdom is secured within the light lineage of all healers.

Women have always been healers. They were the unlicensed doctors and anatomists of Western history. They were abortionists, nurses, and counselors. They were pharmacists, cultivating healing herbs and exchanging secrets of their uses. They were midwives . . . doctors without degrees, barred from books and lectures, learning from each other, and passing on experience from neighbor to neighbor and mother to daughter. They were called "wise women" by the people, witches or charlatans by the authorities. Medicine is part of our heritage as women, our history, our birthright.

BARBARA EHRENREICH & DEIDRE ENGLISH,
Witches, Midwives, and Nurses: A History of Women Healers

The oldest report of a female physician in ancient Egypt is from 2700 BCE. Her name was Merit-Ptah. Both priestesses and priests were also trained as physicians in ancient Egypt; there was no separation between science and spirit. The Kahun papyrus, a medical text from around that time, is thought to have been written for women, as only female healers were permitted to treat women's diseases.[44]

Queen Hatshepsut, the second woman pharaoh of ancient Egypt, supported women physicians in her kingdom and built three medical schools. Her impressive temple at Karnak featured several botanical gardens the priestesses tended.

Cleopatra the physician (not to be confused with the queen) studied with the Greek philosopher Galen and was known for her expert gynecological practice.

Polydamna, a queen and doctor in ancient Egypt, possessed extensive knowledge of the opium poppy and may have trained Helen of Troy (approximately 2000 BCE), who brought the Egyptian medical wisdom to ancient Greece. By the fourth century, it was punishable by death to practice medicine as a woman in ancient Greece, but it was permissible in Egypt around that same time.[45]

In ancient Greece, Agnodice (fourth century BCE), an Athenian physician, attended medical school in disguise and was later put on trial, but granted permission to practice. Women were then given the right to treat other women and children in Greece.

Queen Artemisia of Caria (350 BCE) is thought to be responsible for bringing to light the healing properties of wormwood for numerous diseases.

In Asia, the Chinese Wu were priestesses who danced and drummed into trance, receiving *shen* ("spirits") into their bodies, healing, and prophesying under their inspiration.[46] Yeshe Tsogyal, an important woman in Tibetan Buddhist history, was said to possess powers in bringing people back from the dead.[47]

In Europe throughout the Middle Ages, women practiced as expert herbalists, midwives, surgeons, and nurses.[48] Christianity in the Middle Ages created more danger for women healers, but in some cases they were more protected. Women with special healing talents ran the risk of being accused of witchcraft. In addition to birthing, midwives offered contraception, abortions, and symptom relief. Women were also allowed to practice in convents—one of the few places women were permitted to be formally educated.[49]

Hildegard von Bingen (1098–1179) is known as Germany's first female physician. She was talented in the arts of writing, botany, medicine making, and studying the energetic qualities of plants. Her mystical visions were protected by the church, as they were understood as divinations from God. She also endorsed the use of gemstones, mantras, and hydrotherapy.

Like Hildegard, female royals were able to make extensive contributions in medicine, such as princess and physician Hilda of Whitby, who built an abbey where she practiced and taught medicine. Trota of Salerno is one of the best-known female physicians of the fifth century, and one of the few doctors who advocated better health through diet, exercise, and stress relief. Her writings became an important text, the Trotula, on all manner of female diseases.

Beliefs in witchcraft proliferated in the Middle Ages and Renaissance, making it even more difficult for women to practice medicine. Most people identified as witches were simply skilled at plant medicine and, therefore, considered a threat to the church and aristocracy. "The other side of the suppression of witches as healers was the creation of a new male medical profession, under the protection and

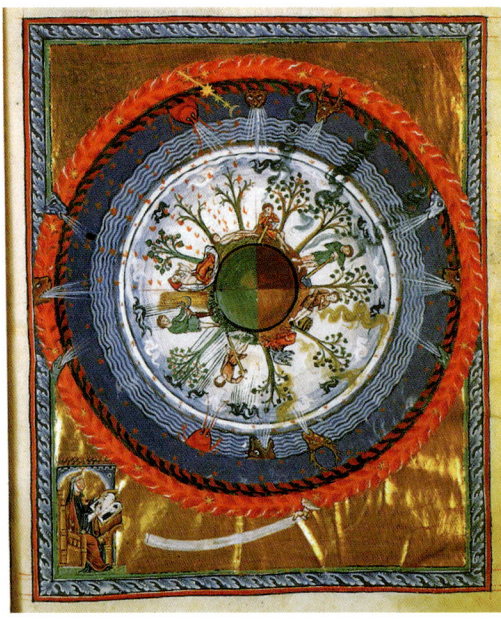

MANDALA
BY HILDEGARD
VON BINGEN

patronage of the ruling classes."[50] Victorian England was marked by increasing oppressive sexual mores, and the pervasive assumption that women were fragile hysterics.[51] As a result, female healers worked mostly undercover, resurfacing again at the turn of the twentieth century, when women, along with BIPOC were finally given the right to a medical education.

In Latin America, curanderas were the predominant folk practitioners of traditional medicine. They were persecuted by the church just as the wise-women healers were in Europe. *Yerberas* focused on herbs, *sobadoras* focused on physical healing, and *parteras* practiced midwifery.[52]

In many parts of pre-colonial Africa, being a woman was commensurate with the art of midwifery. "It wasn't until slavery on the plantation, that women [of color] were appointed as midwives based on their knowledge and familiarity of woman craft."[53] Slave midwives were highly skilled and delivered for white women as well, including the wives of plantation owners.

In North America, many Native American tribes exemplified no gender bias when it came to medicine. There are accounts of both medicine men and women, and "two spirits" people who would have identified as both male and female, or perhaps even as nonbinary.

Harriet Tubman, born Araminta Ross, (circa 1822) is best known for her work in rescuing slaves and bringing them to freedom along the Underground Railroad. Harriet was also a gifted herbalist and nurse who, in addition to healing from her own violent head injury inflicted upon her while trying to protect another slave, was skilled at using herbal root decoctions for soldiers during the Spanish-American War.[54]

A woman is, by nature, a shaman.

CHUCKCHEE PROVERB

EVOLUTION OF THE ASCLEPIUS

Observe the mysterious evolution of the asclepius, also known as the magical staff, possibly originating from the ancient Minoan snake goddess—a feminine figure holding two serpents, perhaps the symbol of Shakti activation (far left). In Ancient Egypt, it is held by Thoth, the god of healing and wisdom. As the symbol travels to Greece, the two serpents become one as is shown with Asclepius, god of knowledge and healing, who studied with Hermes (who held the similar two-serpent caduceus). A recurring theme throughout the alchemical tradition, the serpent here appears with the orphic egg, a symbol of cosmic union. A number of modern medical organizations utilize the asclepius in their logos, including the World Health Organization emblem (far right).

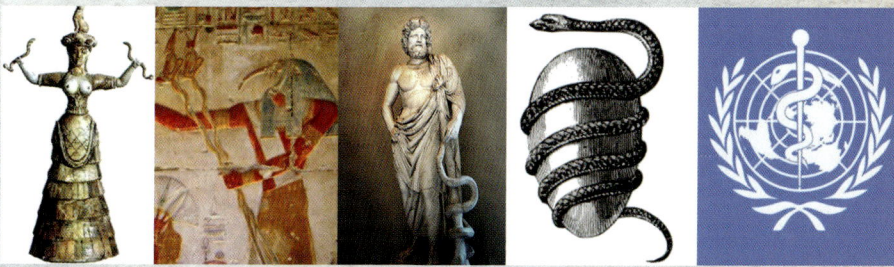

In *Vitalism: The History of Herbalism, Homeopathy, and Flower Essences*, Matthew Wood writes: "The tendency of the magical staff is to drive opposites to the level of complete alienation, and then allow their reconciliation on a higher and more conscious level.... In order to become whole we must differentiate and unite the opposites we find within ourselves."[55]

The Foundations of Flower Essence Therapy

There are several key figures who help us understand the origins and development of contemporary flower essence therapy. While plant medicine was part of every ancient civilization, the roots of flower essence therapy are generally understood as European. As such, no women or people of color are included in the following section, an unfortunate sign of the times.

Paracelsus (1493–1541), born Theophrastus Bombastus von Hohenheim, was a Swiss physician, philosopher, and alchemist who initially worked within the Greek humoral tradition. Far ahead of his time, he possessed knowledge of modern pharmacy, physiology, and biochemistry centuries before they were accepted practice. He may have been one of the first doctors to explore the healing applications of electromagnetic frequencies. He understood the relationship between plants and their environments and worked in accord with that connection. Because of his unorthodox approach and his sometimes mercurial nature, Paracelsus was not accepted by the medical community and spent much of his life wandering in solitude.[56]

While his theories were not accepted by the medical community at the time, his contributions to modern medicine are manifold, and he was also one of the first doctors of his caliber to staunchly oppose the mechanistic nature of conventional medicine during the Middle Ages. He was convinced that healing was both material and spiritual. His revolutionary ideas led him to travel and study ancient alchemy and the subconscious nature of healing. Paracelsus was determined to maintain a connection to Source in his work, and believed health was also connected to the star realm, as astronomy was present throughout many of his writings. In his time, each plant had a corresponding planet. In his water research, Paracelsus would collect the dew from plants during certain planetary transits to observe their energetics.

The idea of the arcana, or secret, underpinning his theories was described using a language of archetypes, a mystical dialect understood by his contemporaries—those versed in the supernatural and astrology. With the arcana, Paracelsus is fully embracing moon consciousness in all its glory: the whole truth is hidden and can only be seen by those initiates who are able to perceive the invisible realms.[57] We also know that he supported women healers, and at one point he burned his text on pharmaceuticals, confessing that he "had learned from the sorceresses all he knew."[58]

Incorporating the spiritual dimension in his work led to many of his discoveries about the microcosm, the macrocosm, the role of the unconscious in physical health, and the subtle bodies. He is recognized as developing the doctrine of signatures, a major component of plant medicine. He believed that all life possessed "a self-regulating and self-healing intelligence."[59] Because of his belief in the vibrational application of medicine, he experimented with dilution, and developed the law of similars, essentially a law of resonance, which would later figure in the development of homeopathy.

Samuel Hahnemann (1755–1843) is best known as the founder of homeopathy. Hahnemann's practice began at a time when medicine was fully aligned with the masculine, with much emphasis on the physical, forceful interventions, "heroic medicine," and the idea that it had to hurt to heal. He took Paracelsus's law of similars and applied it to the curative action of a remedy, believing it was part of universal law—he believed the cure should be similar to the disease. Hahnemann held similar unconventional theories about medicine. The idea that emotional states had anything to do with physical illness was considered preposterous at that time.

While he may not have been outwardly reinforcing Paracelsus's work, he was almost surely informed by the spirit or "vital force" of the plants and minerals he was using. Hahnemann observed the relationship between symptom, remedy, and the aggravation that could arise as a result of the homeopathic preparation working in resonance with an illness. This led him to dilute remedies to an infinitesimal level, and "succus," or shake, the solution in order to potentize it.

Most of Hahnemann's work reflected the simple law of similars; however, later he would develop the concept of chronic miasms. Put simply, these are the underlying causes of all illness that have been passed down energetically from generation to generation since the birth of humankind, possibly from the cosmic beginnings of the Universe. Hahnemann's explanation of the miasms and their link between symptomology and ancestral and cosmic aspects are quite complicated and open to interpretation. In any case, Hahnemann's reinforcement of the vital force, or spirit, in medicine, and the law of similars paved the way for vibrational medicine to advance into future practices.

Rudolf Steiner (1861–1925) was a philosopher, writer, and founder of anthroposophical medicine. He would go on to be one of the key figures in the biodynamic farming movement, as well as the Waldorf education system. He studied under a folk herbalist and held extensive knowledge of plant medicine. Steiner has a slightly different take on science and medicine than the rest of the people in this category, but he is important to mention because many of the tenets of his teachings run parallel to those of flower essence therapy and vibrational medicine.

His work was informed by Goethean science, a branch of study created by Johann Wolfgang von Goethe in eighteenth-century Germany. Goethe developed a phenomenological approach to science (validating unique qualitative experiences) and sought to find a way to properly perceive nature and vital energy and the healing implications of these experiences. He had revolutionary ideas about color, which would eventually reinforce the study of color theory, including demonstrating that we need both light and darkness to perceive color.

Through anthroposophical medicine, Steiner sought to synthesize science and spirituality. He believed the origins of disease lay in the psychic realm. He was inspired by Eastern philosophy, ancient alchemy, mysticism, and various esoterica. In Steiner's mind, we all possess the ability to access other states of consciousness, be clairvoyant, and create any reality we desire by transcending our ego and becoming more conscious.[60] Steiner did lecture on the topics of gender, class, and race, and it should be noted that some of his comments on these topics have been interpreted as less than culturally competent.*[61] Many of his medical findings impacted the work of Dr. Bach and other holistic modalities.

Dr. Edward Bach (1886–1936) was trained as a bacteriologist, immunologist, and later a homeopath. He is the founder of flower essence therapy and the creator of the

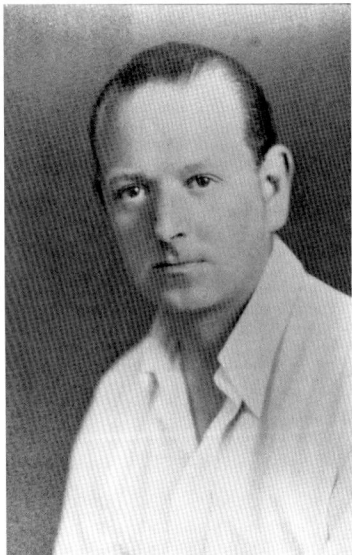

DR. EDWARD BACH. Image courtesy of Julian Barnard.

---

* This is obviously a delicate matter within the Waldorf anthroposophical and biodynamic communities. My current opinion on this is that 1) Steiner wasn't immune to the Euro-American privilege of white males of his time, and some of his comments on gender and race do seem to be problematic; and 2) we should thoroughly acknowledge the blind spots in his teachings in order to learn from them, but not nullify his theories and contributions. It is a both/and situation, not either/or.

original 38 Bach flower remedies, and the Five-Flower Remedy (Rescue Remedy). In his training on the field during World War I, Bach observed that some of his patients would become ill and others wouldn't. He became convinced this was somehow connected to each patient's level of personality and mental and emotional state.

Bach became disenchanted with Western medicine because it addressed the physical results and not the true causes of disease. Also, being a spiritual man, he felt modern science left no room to explain the nonphysical. He felt that physical disease arose from imbalances within the system, from negative thoughts and emotions. He was said to have been highly intuitive, and perhaps even clairvoyant. Inspired by homeopathy and the use of gentle medicine to cure, Bach began to experiment with homeopathic flower preparations to treat both emotional and physical illness. Bach possessed the uncanny ability to see the correspondence of the gesture of the flowers to the gesture (that is, the personality) of people.

Bach credited both Paracelsus and Hahnemann for leading the way, but he felt he needed to expand on their work to make it more accessible to people and connect it back to the natural world. Like Hahnemann, Bach saw that the energetic signature or vital essence of a flower could be captured in water and preserved. He did not, however, apply the principle of "like treats like" in the same way. He felt that a modest amount of poison was not the way to treat disease, "but to balance the negative with the positive, the darkness with the light."[62]

Bach eventually left his career to spend more time in nature and refine his theory around flower medicine. It was during this time that he developed the Twelve Healers, which were twelve essences based exclusively on the psychological state of the patient, ignoring the physical disease. He also published his first text dedicated to flower essences, *Heal Thyself*.[63] According to Bach, each of us has a personality assigned to us at birth, depending on the placement of our natal moon. And that "disease is in itself beneficent, and has for its object the bringing back of the personality to the Divine will of the Soul."[64]

Bach never formally stated which astrological signs corresponded to which plants, for fear of being too dogmatic. I hope Dr. Bach wouldn't mind that I share the following information, as I feel people are ready for the association. This list includes the moon signs suggested by Peter Damian in his book *The Twelve Healers of the Zodiac: The Astrology Handbook of the Bach Flower Therapies*.[65]

Personality	Plant	Astrological Sign
Tormented	Agrimony	Sagittarius
Terror	Rock Rose	Scorpio
Fear	Mimulus	Capricorn
Indifference	Clematis	Pisces
Pain	Impatiens	Aries
Indecision	Scleranthus	Libra
The Enthusiast	Vervain	Leo
Discouragement	Gentian	Taurus
The Doormat	Centaury	Virgo
The Fool	Cerato	Gemini
Grief	Water Violet	Aquarius
Congestion	Chicory	Cancer

Bach would go on to create twenty-five additional flower essences and one unique environmental essence, rock water. Bach was thinking bigger than merely curing disease. He was called to assist people in attaining deep equilibrium with themselves, others, and the entire macrocosm. He felt that "health depends on being in harmony with our souls"[66] and that true healing must come from the spiritual level, then reach to the emotional/mental, and lastly connect with the physical body. He was aware that each of us arrives on Earth with a personality, and that it was possible to transcend this egoic reality and exist in alignment with our higher selves. Disease was a result of disharmony between soul (heart) and mind (ego).

Bach was very clear on the origin of the species of plants he used. He was sensitive to making remedies in the plants' native environments, as was the case with vine and olive, which were produced in the Mediterranean region. He realized that part of the medicine involved honoring the environment where the plant lived.

With the help of Nora Weeks, his partner, Dr. Bach's legacy lives on by way of his teachings and remedies, which are still produced according to his ritual and specifications at his garden at the Bach Centre in Wallingford, England.

Color Theory and Rainbow Consciousness

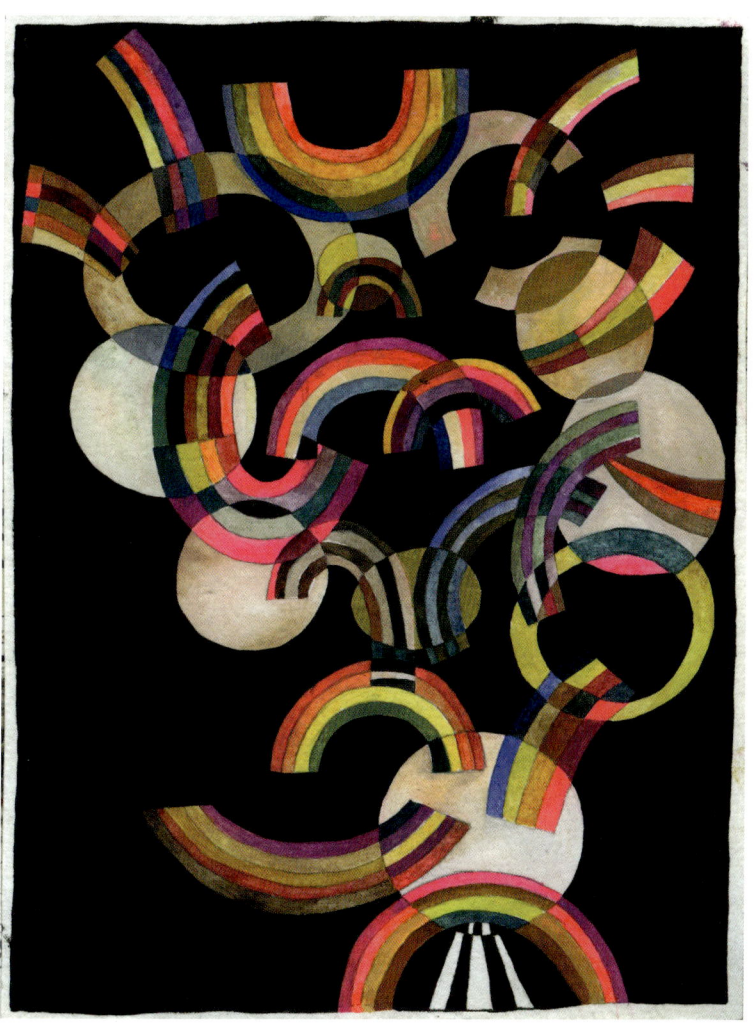

I've always had a fascination with rainbows and have met many people who feel similarly connected to them. The spectrum of the rainbow and light are connected to the great mystery and beauty of the devic kingdom of the flowers. Historically, all natural phenomena seemed to play a role in the world's varying creation mythologies. Rainbows were regarded differently in various cultures, and the materialization of one was generally interpreted as a significant natural occurrence. In Norse mythology, the rainbow was perceived as a conduit between Earth and the heavens. Similarly, the Celtic tradition revered rainbows as highly auspicious and believed a pot of gold could be found at the end of one with the help of a leprechaun from the faerie realm. Rainbows were commonly seen as a blessing and sign of abundance in much classical Christian art, as shown in depictions of the tale of Noah and his ark. In Homer's *Iliad*, Iris was the goddess of the rainbow, and she was a messenger of the gods. The Australian Aboriginals believed that the creator of all life was a rainbow serpent. In the Tibetan Buddhist tradition, when a particularly evolved soul leaves the physical body in death, it travels into nirvana and passes into the state of the rainbow body, or *jalu powa chemo*. Their bodies literally turn to rainbow light, a phenomenon that has been observed and recorded throughout history.[67]

The rainbow has become the sign of solidarity within the LGBTQ community as a colorful symbol of inclusivity and diversity. According to Doreen Virtue, "Rainbow Children" who are incarnating now hold Buddha and Christ consciousness.[68] Rainbow spectrums occur other places in nature, for instance when we look inside an abalone a shell or a quartz crystal.

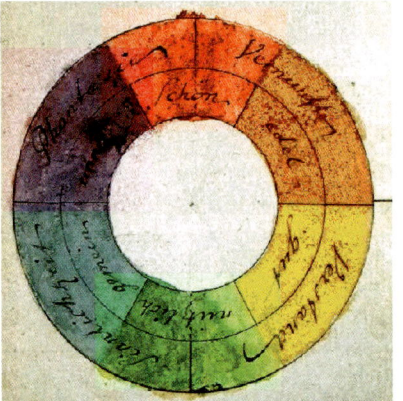

GOETHE'S COLOR WHEEL, 1810

After Newton suggested his ideas on color theory, in the beginning of the nineteenth century, Johann Wolfgang von Goethe offered an opposing opinion that color was observable. Goethe disagreed with Newton's theory of colors and was more interested in the subjective experience of color. He felt that color was the "resolution of the tension between light and dark" and one needed both shadow and light to perceive color.[69] Goethe offered some general distinctions between color and emotion; for example, yellow is "brightness, serene, gay, softly exciting."[70] Bach created mustard essence (from the bright yellow flower) for the depression that descends out of the blue.

Much of our experience of color depends on our ability to perceive it—it's highly subjective, just like our perception of plants. We naturally connect our soul experience to color; for example, seeing red, feeling blue, being green with envy. Color is one of the dominant features in flowers, and so understanding the relationship between vibrational states and flower colors is valuable. According to Patricia Kaminski, color is alive, a living aspect of a plant.[71] Rudolf Steiner suggested there are more colors between indigo and blue that we're still evolving to be able to see. And this is true: there are many colors that exist beyond the bandwidth of frequencies that we can physically see. Wavelengths are measurements of light, which are also necessary to consider when perceiving color.

Flowers hold a special connection to the color spectrum and the rainbow. Of course, there are colors in all parts of the plant: root, seed, stem, leaf, and bark; however, flowers are the part of the plant that are distinguished as the agents of color. In the words of Ayurvedic herbalist Anne McIntyre, "It is the flower that displays itself in all its magnificence, not only to attract pollinating insects, but also to bring its healing nature to the attention of mankind who has such need of its gifts."[72] Before flowers existed, the world contained far less color, and was mostly green, gray, brown, and blue.[73] So, the rainbow spectrum also corresponds to evolution and ecological diversity because they are intrinsically linked. It would be overly simplistic to assign a generalized formula of each color and its characteristics (such as red equals love, or blue equals intuition), as colors mean different things to different groups. But there are significant overlapping interpretations of the relationship between color, emotion, plant signature, and indication. This goes for the chakra system, too, which corresponds to the rainbow spectrum.

That a person's etheric field could emanate a rainbow spectrum is quite an abstract concept to us in the West, especially if you're still skeptical of the validity of the subtle bodies and energy. However, for many of us who study and perceive energy, a layer of color is as real and discernable as any physical quality. Like vibratory states, each color has a vibration, a measurable frequency.[74] In this way, color serves as both a measurement and a subjective, perceptual aspect to understand energy and flowers. All colors of the rainbow are necessary for the complete spectrum. And, interestingly, how we are evolving to see color is changing, as evidenced by the recent addition of magenta into our material world, despite its abundant representation in flowers, especially in tropical regions. Each ray has its place and purpose within the evolutionary journey, physically and spiritually. (If you feel a connection between color and the chakra system, I would highly recommend *Eastern Body, Western Mind: Psychology and the Chakra System as a Path to the Self* by Anodea Judith.)

I have been carefully recording notes on color characteristics over the years. If you feel a connection to color, this is a useful way into working with flower medicine. The following is a list I have compiled that includes some suggested essences for the particular characteristics:

- Red—passion, intensity, heat, upward moving, fire, earth, warning, survival, blood, rootedness, root chakra; Woodland Essence's red Trillium, which provides centeredness during cycles of life such as death and rebirth
- Orange—energetic, warming, outward moving, sexuality, relationships, sacral chakras
- Yellow—joy, sun, light, youth, confidence, outward moving, bile, solar plexus chakra, confidence, will; chamomile for easing tension in the solar plexus
- Green—calm, cool, nature, love, compassion, forgiveness, courage, heart chakras
- Blue—calming, space, nervous system, water, air, cooling, downward moving, communication, throat chakra; blue vervain
- Violet—spirituality, intuition, psychic abilities, wisdom, third-eye chakra
- Magenta—the beginning and the ending, vitality, Echinacea; star realm, shooting star
- Pink—love, nurturing
- White—purity, neutrality, bones; angelica, for connection to the angelic realm and one of my most-used protection essences

- Brown—first chakra issues; chocolate lily, for aversion to digestive and reproductive functions of the body
- Black—the shadow, death and rebirth; center of borage is black and points to its use for depression

EXERCISE | Rainbow Worksheet

If one construct of the modern world is a black-and-white binary, then the rainbow epitomizes the multidimensional opposite. Here's a chart for you to fill in with your own impressions of the rainbow spectrum. What does each color evoke in you? See if you can tune in to any felt senses. Jot down a few words that come up for each ray.

BLACK
RED
ORANGE
YELLOW
GREEN
BLUE
INDIGO
VIOLET
WHITE
MAGENTA
BROWN

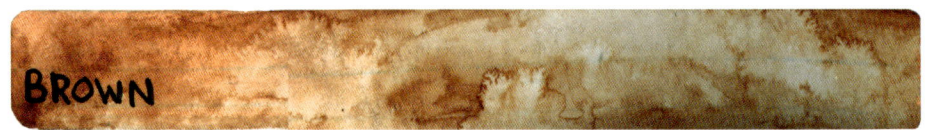

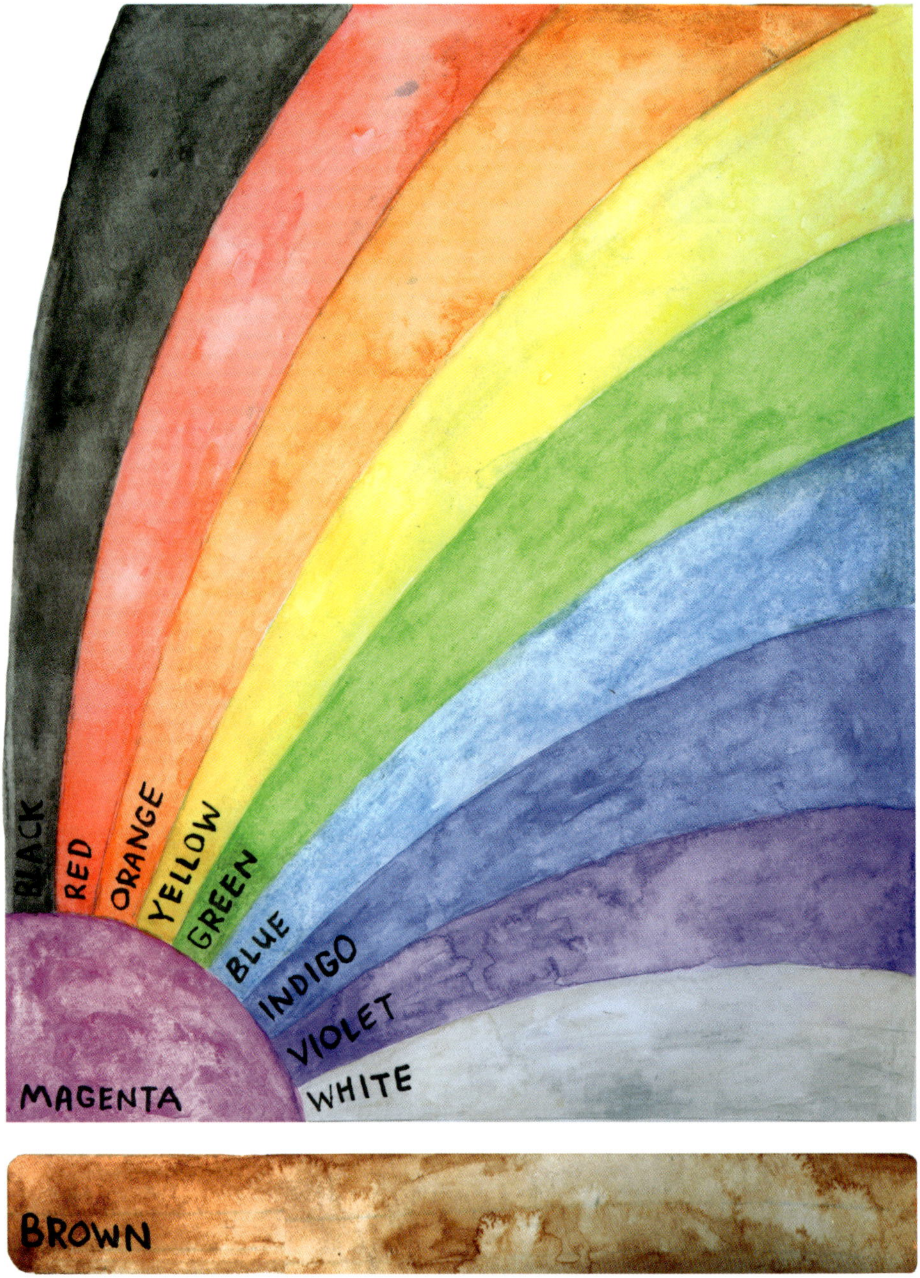

The Flower of Life

The flower of life is a sacred symbol that can be found in many ancient texts, and in artwork and architecture from around the world. There is great mystery and speculation about the meaning of this symbol. To me, like the rainbow, it represents the connection to our ancestors, the divine, and all life. It illustrates the mystery of life and all that we can't define, the wisdom in not knowing. The circle itself being such a supreme symbol of unity and wholeness, it then multiplies in meaning with its many interlocking circles, to create an elegant pattern of interconnectivity. It contains many mathematical codes that serve as the building blocks to understanding many theories of physics, chemistry, and biology. Geometrically, it contains the tree of life, which in kabbalah represents the origin of all life. It is thought that the dimensions of Stonehenge correspond with the symbol. Leonardo da Vinci studied the flower of life and its relationship to other geometric theories such as the golden ratio. Observed three dimensionally, you can see the merkaba and the structure of the tetrahedron, or pyramid. In the alchemical tradition, Metatron's cube, which was formed out of the flower of life, represented the five platonic solids that create a template for all creation.

FLOWER OF LIFE

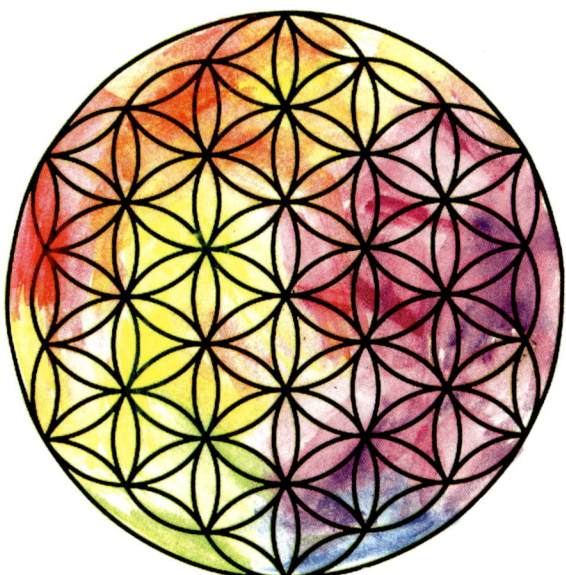

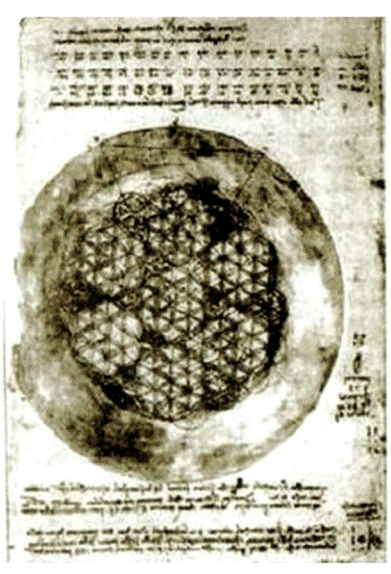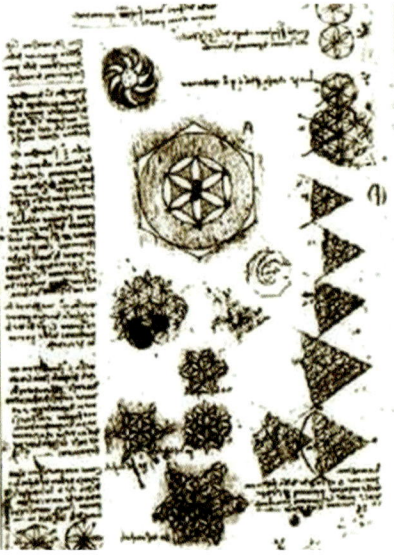

DA VINCI'S SKETCHES
of the flower of life.

The oldest known example of the flower of life can be found at the Osirion, a temple dedicated to Osiris, at Abydos in Egypt. I had the privilege of visiting this site in 2010, and saw with my own eyes the perfectly executed symbols on a giant granite slab. It wasn't painted or etched, and it is unknown how the inscription was produced. These massive pieces of granite, some weighing an estimated fifty tons, had somehow been transported hundreds of miles from the nearest quarry where this particular stone could be found. Then, they were perfectly cut into square pillars and hoisted up and stacked onto one another. The precision of the symbols is shockingly accurate. How could this have been accomplished thousands of years ago?

In Abydos, it felt as if the flower of life was showing me the infinite potentials of healing and reality, beyond what I knew was possible. Looking back, I see that this sacred symbol was heralding a new path for me. After returning home from Egypt, I left New York and my old career to go back to school and study counseling. Nowadays, the flower of life comes to me synchronistically and in dreams and meditations, like a beacon of hope when I need it most. I can spot it in nature, especially within flowers of the Asteraceae (daisy) family. It's always revealing more information to me in other formats, such as stones, artwork, and music. Again and again, it reminds me the mystery of life is continually unfolding around us, guiding us into subtler and subtler realities.

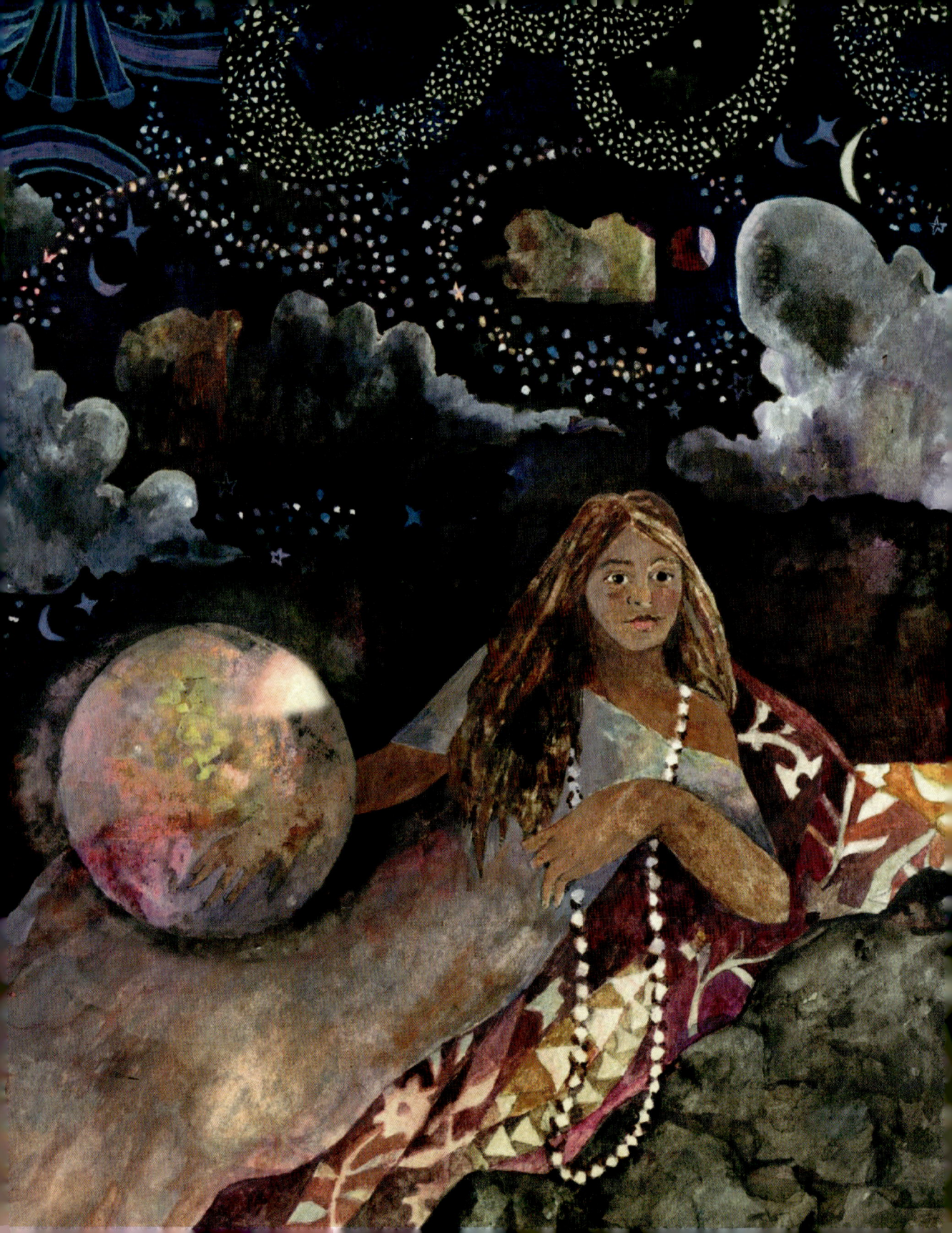

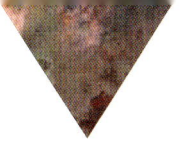

CHAPTER FOUR

Flower Rituals for Healing and Transformation

A RITUAL IS ANY PRACTICE you perform with intention. Like the symbol of the rainbow, rituals connect the physical world with the nonphysical plane and provide more ways for us to enact our dreams and potentials. Flower essences work so powerfully with ritual because they work at highly subtle, refined levels—at the level of spirit. Rituals work in a similar frequency, with the energy of intention, prayer, affirmation, and offering. Because ritual engages the spirit or energetic level of your practice, flower essences are perfectly attuned to support this type of work.

Rituals are intentional practices that connect me more intimately with myself, with others, with my ancestors and guides, with nature, and with Spirit. They help engender greater trust within my own heart wisdom. This book owes much to the ritual I created around writing, wherein I would ground, pray, and take a flower essence before sitting down to compose. Engaging in ritual work is a way to give back beyond the level of self: you can offer a ritual for a group of people, a place, to animals that might need your prayers, or even the elements, like a sacred body of water. Rituals can serve as potent ceremonies to support healing change on both astral and physical levels, when a physical intervention is not possible—for example, prayer for an interpersonal conflict when dialogue isn't an option. Some are part of my daily routines, such as my morning meditation. Others are more infrequent, such as the New Year's Day (according to Gregorian calendar) ceremony my partner and I do together in Vermont. There are days of the year that are important for me to honor with rituals, such as full and new moons, solstices and equinoxes, birthdays, anniversaries, and death days. Ritual is not only a significant part of my healing and medicine-making practice—it actually becomes part of the energetic signature of my medicine. My ritual prayer is part of every client session. The more my healing practices deepen, the more I trust in the transformative power of my rituals and in the ceremonies of, and with, others.

The ancient world was steeped in rituals—they were highly sensory experiences, of which plants and flowers played a significant role. Historically, rituals have been used to honor certain energies, gods and goddesses, holy people, natural phenomena, initiations, and transitions such as birth and death. They were closely related to all aspects of life. Specific days and ceremonies were set aside for protecting the crops and giving thanks for the harvest. Sacred rituals were the practices employed by the initiates of the mystery schools to access greater levels of consciousness.

When we discuss ritual, we are delving into ancient traditions and, therefore, must be sensitive to cultural appropriation. If you are in a position of reaping financial gain from certain borrowed rituals, a fair energetic compensation should be a consideration. Some questions to consider: Are you borrowing practices from other cultures? Are you borrowing plants from other places? What are some rituals connected to your ancestry? If you are using plants or practices from cultures other than your own, are you offering appropriate credit for them?

An irony about white settlers is that, while we adopted and co-opted many indigenous practices, many of us are cut off from our own cultural traditions. In some cases, white people were both the colonized and the colonizers. Colonization removed the spiritual aspect of all traditional practices. We are spiritual beings; we innately want a connection to the spirit world. How we arrive at that connection should be especially thoughtful of those groups and traditions that hold the wisdom we are seeking. I have to wonder: at what point do all our roots become indigenous? Learning more about one's heritage can be an awesome way to feel a connection to those practices that are part of who you are and where you came from. As noted earlier, I have always felt a deep kinship with the folklore of the British Isles, and one day hope to spend more time in this area researching my family roots. In the meantime, I enjoy learning about certain foods and recipes that were traditionally used during the wintertime holidays.

My relationship to rituals has changed over the years as I've reevaluated what my relationship to the idea of ritual is. What does ritual mean to you? Many of us are indoctrinated into rituals that we feel little to no connection with. And perhaps these are possible ways into greater connection. My partner and I don't have children; however, there are parts of Christmas I want to enjoy and honor, even though it seems so focused on kids and consumerism. I want us to be consciously creating our own traditions instead of blindly going along with whatever. So now, we are committed to making holiday cards together. We will bring back some greenery from Vermont and cook a holiday dinner. In this way, we are consciously choosing how we participate in certain traditions and rituals and creating greater coherence and connection with them. Are there any rituals you feel connected to? Are there some you feel less connected to? What are some ways you could create more of a conscious connection to them? Every culture has its own traditions and magical practices.

This chapter will offer more context around rituals, especially connected to the moon, and creative ways to integrate them into your own practices. People seek out my help because they would like to connect with their spiritual selves and cultivate a spiritual practice. Rituals are a big part of this cultivation. However you are guided to pray and practice, this is your own, unique medicine, and you can trust that this is a natural way to heal. One of the lessons of the moon is to learn to trust our intuition. Allow her to guide you to explore in your rituals. Working in the flow of natural rhythms, connecting with our tribes, celebrating and honoring life and death, and making medicine are all parts of moon ritual wisdom.

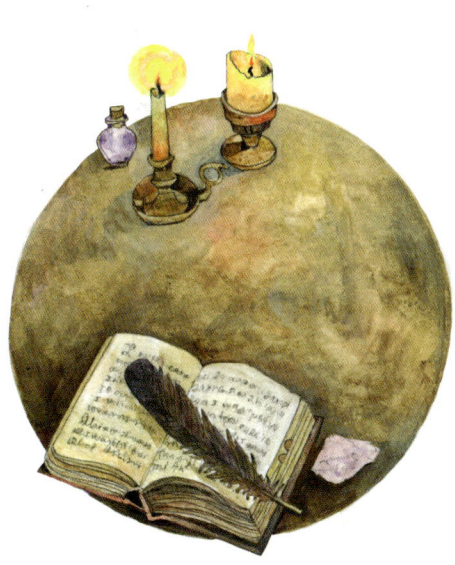

I highly recommend creating a space of your own, sometimes referred to as an altar, to cultivate this work. It could be connected to your apothecary, or in a separate area. Your altar is a private sanctuary for your ritual and spiritual work. Some elements it could include are a candle, any sacred objects, flowers, stones, shells, leaves; or pictures of people, ancestors, animals, or places that are very important to you. It can be very simple. You may keep a protective or clearing flower essence there such as yarrow or moxa, or make a protective mist. The etymology of the word *altar* is to "raise up," so think of your altar as a living space of peace, potential, and magic. The more time you spend cultivating your spiritual practice in your healing space, the more you will harness and ground the energy into a powerful practice.

RITUAL | Re-Centering

In between seeing clients, I have a few simple rituals I utilize to re-center myself. When I do this, I know my clients can feel a difference too. It's a way for me to be totally clear and present for people, and I consider it to be part of offering a high level of care. If you work in a service-oriented profession, you might want to consider creating an easy practice around re-centering. You may want to take a single flower essence such as FES's sagebrush, or a blend such as Alaskan Essences' Soul Support or Delta Gardens' Clearing. Flower essence mists are also a great option to use in spaces either before, after, or in between healing work. A ritual for creating your own protective mist can be found on page 135.

1. *Close your eyes and ground your energy in a few deep breaths.*

2. *Visualize your aura/subtle bodies (I see mine like an egg-shaped orb) and clear it/them with cobalt-blue light. Visualize anything that might be stuck to your aura, or weighing you down, gently falling to the Earth. We're just gently clearing the aura here.*

3. *Breathe into your heart and your root chakras. Feel that sense of inner alignment coming back into your center point.*

4. *Say to yourself, silently or out loud, a centering mantra such as, "I am here. I am open. I am clear. I am in perfect alignment."*

The History of Flowers in Healing Traditions

Flowers played a substantial role in ancient healing traditions. Flowers are the part of the plant that evolved to be in relationship with its environment. Evolutionarily, angiosperms, or flowering plants, evolved later in history, signifying the higher level of consciousness of inflorescence. All plants grow toward the sun; however, this ascending energy is more focused in the flower.[1] It is estimated that flowers emerged around 250 million years ago; without them, human life would not be possible.[2] Our ancestors experienced plants as living beings; their communication with the plant spirit, or devic kingdom, was sacrosanct, and has been passed down through ancient healing traditions, art, literature, and folklore. All parts of the plant were used for healing, and all parts of the flower were celebrated for their therapeutic applications: their beauty, their physical sensation, their scent, and their energetic properties.

The following are some examples of how flowers were used and regarded throughout history.

The Nile River is said to be the cradle of civilization, evoking imagery of a lush Eden. The lotus (both blue and white varieties) is one of the earliest flowers to be depicted here. Reliefs and paintings frequently adorned the walls of the temples. The essential oil was used in rites for birth, celebration, and death. Egyptians associated the white lotus with creation. The Egyptians adored flowers, which is evident by their abundant depiction in the ancient art and texts. They were skilled herbalists and grew impressive gardens that were sources of medicinal plants, food, and plants for rites, celebrations, and pleasure. Tree branches, such as acacia, were also used during rituals and celebrations. Trees were thought to have particular relationship to the neteru, and many temples featured specific trees for each god or goddess.[3]

PROCESSION OF EGYPTIAN WOMEN

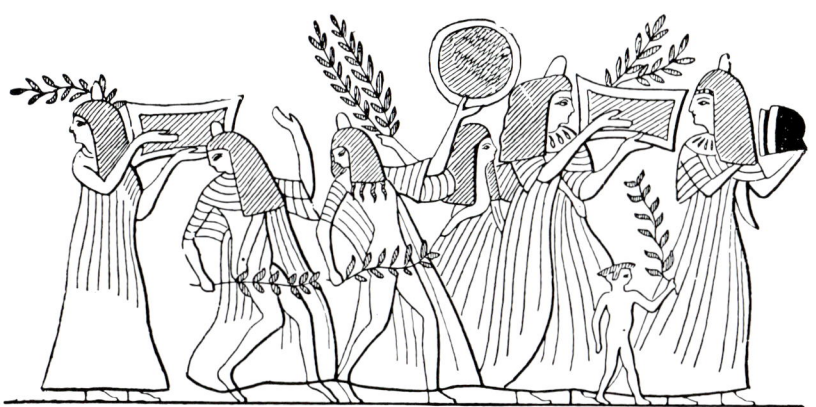

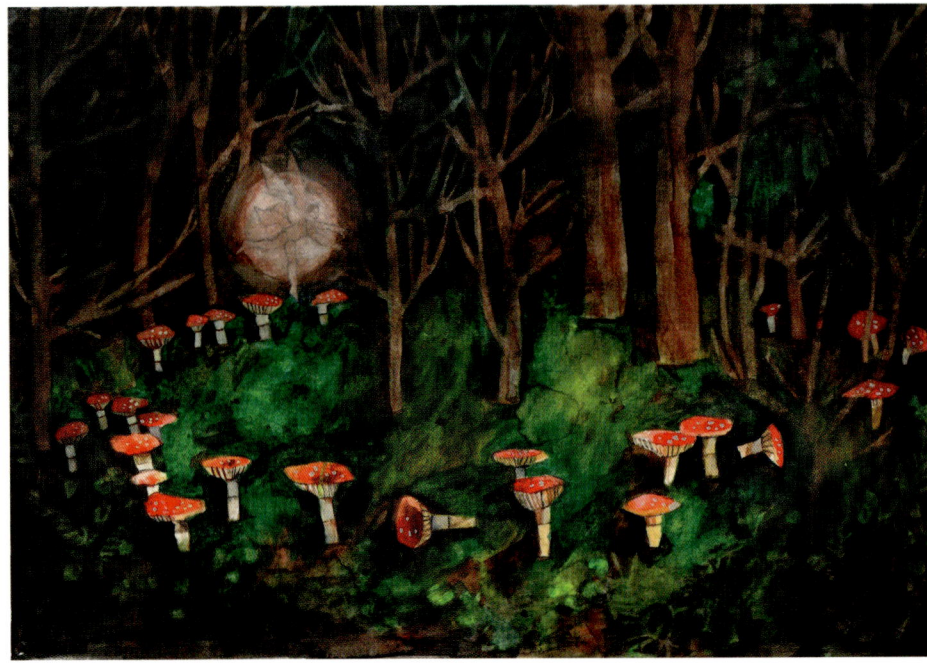

FAERIE RING. Faerie rings are naturally occurring and are said to be portals to the realm of the fae.

The ancient Egyptians were highly ritualistic in their funerary rites. Multiple garlands and collars of leaves and flowers such as the blue lotus, olive, willow, and cornflower were placed on the mummies for burial. The deceased were surrounded by flowers as they embarked on their journey to the underworld. Wreaths were also worn as crowns for their aesthetic beauty, their scent, and their connection to the divine. Flowers were given as gifts and offerings to deities. White flowers were often a symbol of purity.

The Greeks and Romans adopted the Egyptian tradition of wearing flower crowns. Maidens wore white flower crowns to signify their virtue. Laurel halos were worn as a sign of respect by military victors. Aphrodite gave a red rose to her son, Eros, which came to be associated with romantic love.[4]

Artemis, the moon goddess of ancient Greece, revived the flowers at night with dew and then her brother, Apollo, gave the sun's rays to the plants in the daytime.[5]

In ancient China, women wore orange blossom flowers in their wedding crowns to symbolize fertility.

Throughout Europe in the Middle Ages, the quest for the holy grail was the attempt at harnessing the powers of the tree of life, which was portrayed as a blossom.

In the British Isles, wells and springs were considered sacred and were decorated with flowers in springtime. This part of the world is also home to rich faerie lore. Foxgloves were worn by the "little folks", bluebells were thought to ring when fairies were gathering, eating primroses allowed one to see faeries, St. John's wort was used as protection against spells, ragwort was used by faeries for horses, cowslip flowers were used to find faerie gold, and the four-leaf clover could break a faerie spell.[6]

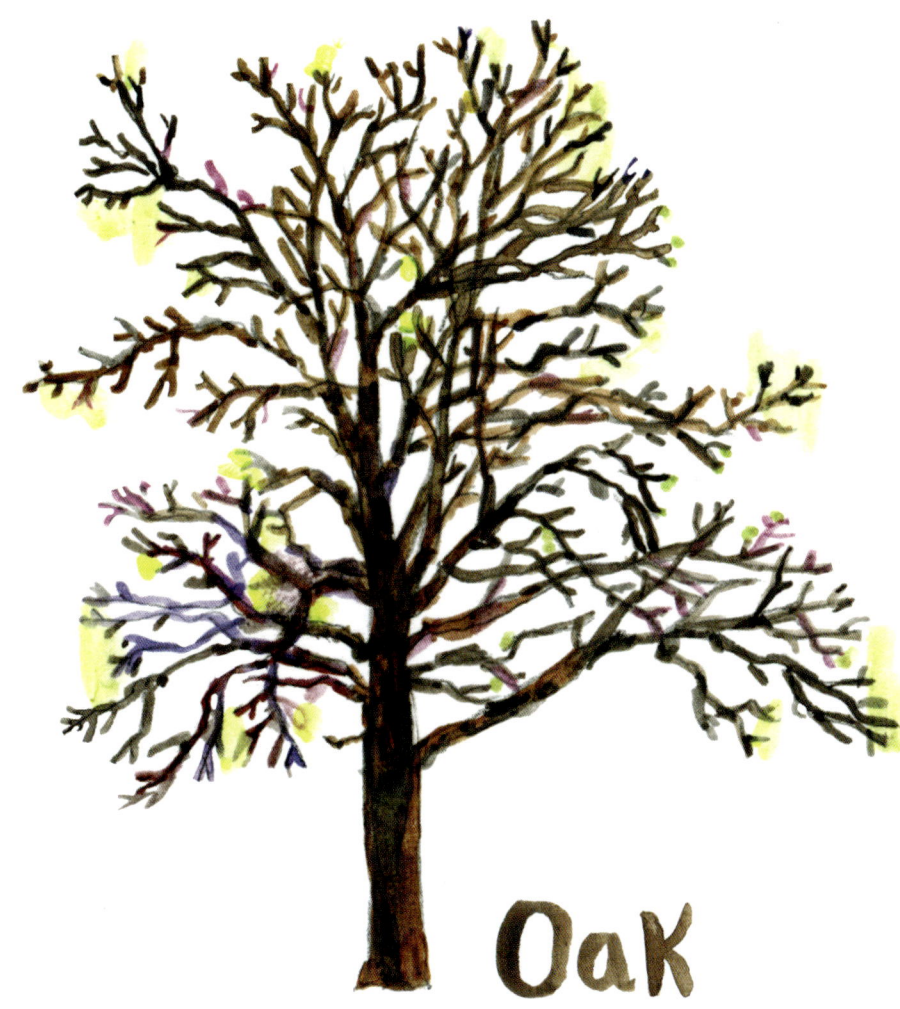

QUERCUS ROBUR. Celtic plant lore is very connected to the elemental and plant spirits. Druids created their language from trees, most notably the oak and the holly. Flowers and berries of the trees were thought to contain especially magical properties.

Oak
Quercus robur

The mythology from this time also celebrates tree medicine, especially from the hazel, alder, elder, oak, birch, ash, and hawthorn.[7]

Mayan and Incan traditions in Central and South America utilized spiritual bathing, essentially bathing with plants and flowers for a variety of psycho-spiritual emotional disturbances.[8]

In India and Bangladesh, Hindu deities are honored with floral garlands, as are newlyweds. A particular group in India, known as Sattarars, are holy people who never

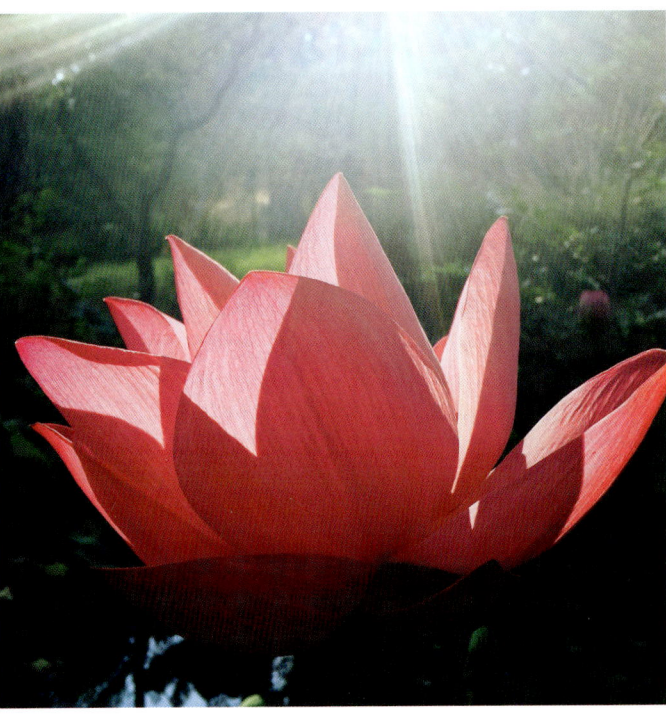

PINK LOTUS AT TERRA FLORA.
summer 2016.

marry and dedicate their lives to the art of garland making. In India, the lotus has always been a spiritual allegory of transformation, associated with the goddess Lakshmi.

Buddhist tradition honors the water lily and lotus as symbols of enlightenment as they bloom out of the mud.

In North America, the Comanche believed the lupine sprang up, despite the selfishness of humans, to remind us to love. The Ojibwa named the yellow lady's slipper after Koo-Koo-Lee, a medicine woman who sacrificed her life to find medicine in the woods to save her husband. The mayflower, or trailing arbutus, is the flower of the Odawa people. This fragrant flower is represented by a loving maiden in whose footsteps the beautiful flowers grow.

Floriography, "the language of flowers," became popular during Victorian times as a way to communicate otherwise taboo messages through individual or mixed flower arrangements. Herbalist, naturopath, and flower essence practitioner Julia Graves feels that floriography should not be confused with the doctrine of signatures, rather "a secret code between two parties in a rigid, moralistic society."[9]

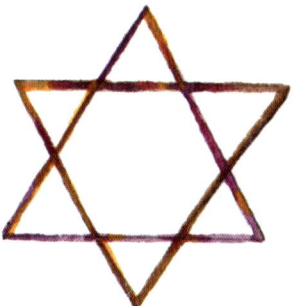

Safety, Protection, and Psychic Hygiene

In the last chapter, we discussed the necessity for safety when utilizing flower essences. Here again, let's consider the role of safety in ritual, along with protection and psychic hygiene. I'm speaking of safety and protection within a mostly energetic context here because more awareness around these topics is valuable for us to know when working with flower essences and vibrational medicine.

We exist in a world filled with duality, and this extends into some of the invisible realms as well. It is not all light and love in the physical and nonphysical realms. If we are seeking to raise our vibration, then it makes sense to be discerning about the energies we are both projecting into the world and those we are exposing ourselves to. Other people, places, and thought forms are three of the main sources of psychic intrusion. The energetic fields around these can have deleterious effects on our health, especially for the highly empathic. You may be absorbing negativity, which can manifest as fatigue, confusion, nightmares, anxiety, depression, and repetitive thoughts that don't feel like they were generated by you, but by an external influence.

Many times, when we introduce light into our lives, there is a shadow force that accompanies it as a natural cosmic balance. This is not a bad thing—merely a law of our Universe. And while light attracts light, when we call in energies and open ourselves up to other realms and realities, we are also vulnerable to attracting darker energies, even if our intention is for light and good. I've found that density, in urban areas especially, can be quite taxing for some people. It is necessary to take protective measures, especially at the beginning stages of spiritual travels.

Again, balance is the operative state for being in alignment. When we are in alignment, we can most easily discern what energy (emotions, thoughts, projections) are not ours, but are perhaps connected to someone else, the collective, or even the past. We can see where we are getting hooked into energies that are pulling us out of balance. For instance, when we are in alignment, toxic personalities tend to avoid us, and we are less susceptible to addictive behaviors. This is the same with toxic energy: it will find another source to hook into. The more time we spend in alignment, the more we can reset our natural baseline and become more naturally resilient and discerning.

For those of us in helping and professional healing roles, we need to be extra careful with ourselves. This is especially true for those involved in healing and transformational justice activism, as burnout can be especially high. Much like professional runners wouldn't want to exhaust themselves before a big race, helpers must attend to their energy and subtle bodies as well as their physical health. If we choose to integrate healing justice into the intentions around our ritual work, we magnify the mission of healing justice, which is "both a paradigm and a set of practices that invites practitioners to heal themselves at the same time that they heal the world."[10]

Healing work naturally attracts empaths. An empath is someone who is especially sensitive to stimuli: both physical and subtle. They may have experiences deemed supernatural by Western standards, and that could be challenging to make sense of and integrate. Empaths possess many gifts that make them naturally attuned to helping, such as possessing heightened abilities for perceiving the emotional patterns in people and groups. Many empaths are trauma survivors and are sometimes more vulnerable to emotional toxicity and psychic bonding.

On an energetic level, recognizing that these patterns aren't personal, but merely an energetic exchange, can be helpful in healing from toxic relationships and situations. Rituals can serve to strengthen the subtle bodies, or auric field, from psychic attack, and fortify the whole self. They can also be used to honor work that has been done, teachings that have been integrated, and cords that are ready to be severed in order to move on with one's life in a healthier way.

These techniques require practice. The more consistent time and energy you offer your protective practices, the more you will feel their beneficial effects. With the advent of technology, we are seeing an unknown number of electromagnetic frequencies (EMFs) entering our world. Many of us feel that these increased frequencies directly correlate to an increase in disease, and protection rituals serve as a barrier and counterbalance to EMFs. Once you begin regularly utilizing a clearing practice in your home, for instance, you will likely feel the difference. My partner and I are so sensitive that now we do some kind of home purifying once a week.

RITUAL | Creating a Protective Mist

I love using flower essences in mist form for my home and office. I go through a lot of mists as I use them during sessions, between clients, when I get home, and when I clear our home, so making my own is also practical.

For this ritual, you will need a glass bottle and mist nozzle. You may work with either store-bought essences, ones you've wildcrafted yourself, or both. You can select one or a few of the essences from the accompanying list, if you aren't sure what to use. I like to add a few drops of essential oil as well, such as rose, neroli, or violet.

1. *Ground your energy and say your prayer (if you have one). Ask for permission to connect with the spirits of the plants you are calling on. Call on the spirit of divine protection to be part of your ritual.*

2. *Fill the mist bottle up with 70 percent spring water and 30 percent brandy.*

3. *Add a few drops of essential oil to the bottle.*

4. *Add the flower essences you've selected. (Three drops of stock essence per half ounce of water and brandy solution).*

5. Close the bottle and swirl three times clockwise and three times counterclockwise, while asking for the remedy to be purified and blessed. I also ask that it be of the highest potency, used for the highest good, and the highest healing.

Beginner Essences for Inviting Grounding, Safety, and Protection

Flower Essence Producer Abbreviations:

Alaskan Essences = AE

Bach Essences = BE

Delta Gardens = DG

Flower Essence Society = FES

Bloesem Remedies Nederlands = BR

Woodland Essence = WE

A number of these flowers can be found in old *materia medica* (list of remedies) as they have historically been used for protection across many cultures throughout history:

AE Soul Support—a blend of cattail pollen, chalice well, cotton grass, fireweed, Labrador tea, malachite, river beauty, ruby, and white fireweed; brings strength and stability during emergencies, stress, trauma, and transformation, while providing support to rejuvenate and restore balance on all levels.

AE Guardian—a blend of covelite, devil's club, round-leaf orchid, stone circle, white violet, and yarrow; helps you create a powerful forcefield of protection in your aura. It invokes positive, harmonious energies that help you claim your energetic space, maintain your grounding, and feel the protection of strong, healthy boundaries.

BR Protection Combination Essence—a combination of sneezewort, greater celandine, rue, and sensitive weed; surrounds and protects you with light; restorative.

FES, DG, or BR angelica—ability to contact spiritual realms on the soul level; to feel help from higher, beneficent forces.

FES mountain pennyroyal—protection against negative programming and psychic bonding.

FES Yarrow Environmental Protection—a blend of white, pink, and golden yarrow, Echinacea, herbal tinctures of yarrow and Echinacea, and sea salt; strengthens and protects against toxic environmental influences, geopathic stress, and other hazards of technology-dominated modern life. This includes the disruptive effects of radiation on human energy fields from X-rays, televisions, computer monitors, electromagnetic fields, airplane flights, and nuclear fallout.

FES pink yarrow—for appropriate emotional boundaries; overly absorbent auric field; dysfunctional merging with others.

DG Protection Set—angelica, cinquefoil, garlic, pennyroyal, rue, St. John's wort, yarrow; protection blend of all seven essences.

DG red cedar—offers stability, wisdom, and rootedness during times of turbulence.

DG or FES rue—repels negativity directed towards us by others; containment of psychic forces.

Relaxation is another useful strategy in helping one to feel safe and grounded. Here is a list of some of my favorite essences to encourage a more calm state.

Flower Essences That Encourage Relaxation

BE red chestnut—"the cutting-free flower," from symbiosis to autonomy. Develops the soul's potential for caring and having compassion for others, having a calm and serene disposition when considering the situation of others or life events; for obsessive fear and apprehension about the well-being of others.

BE cherry plum—"the openness flower," from overload to relaxation; develops the soul's potential for composure.

BE Impatiens—"the time flower," from impatience to patience; develops the soul's potential for patience and gentleness.

DG dandelion—relaxes anxiety in muscles, for when anger can inhibit relaxation.

DG borage—gives peace, lightness, and courage; brings relief to burden, depression, or melancholy.

DG lemon balm—produces a calm which allows deeper exploration or work; one's mind remains keen while enveloped by peacefulness; useful in combination with remedies which serves as a catalyst for movement or a stirring of emotion.

DG golden amaranthus—learning to let go of overcontrol; becoming aware of the power of the higher self; tuning into the ease of life; developing ways to flow with the currents; eases transitions.

FES California valerian—positive qualities: tranquility and inner equilibrium; inner confidence for the future due to the soul's understanding of prior experiences; peaceful acceptance of life experiences; patterns of imbalance: shallow breathing due to anxiety about the future, nervous agitation or insomnia, worry and unease when facing future life events that are viewed as challenging.

FES chamomile—letting go of nervousness and emotional tension; difficulty in sleeping, insomnia; especially good for children.

FES lavender—calming overstimulated nerves; nervous or high-wired energy states; depletion of physical forces; insomnia.

WE wild rose—assists one in finding a healthy balance between activity and relaxation; for those who try to over-form their lives; adds a sense of relaxing into the essence of the moment.

Grounding

Grounding is the practice of sending one's subtle energies down into, and connecting with, the Earth. The Earth possesses its own electrical field, and if you lie, sit, or walk on the ground, you actually connect with the frequency of it. The Earth's frequency has a measurement of 432 hertz, also known as the Schumann resonance. Just as nature heals, the effects of spending time grounding or "earthing" have been empirically validated as reducing inflammation, lowering stress, and improving wound healing.[11] While the effects can be enhanced if you can connect directly with the Earth, grounding is the practice of accessing the Earth energy anywhere, regardless of geographic location or ability level. Grounding has taken on a huge role in my practices and rituals. It's the first thing I do before I see a client, have a difficult conversation, teach a class, make medicine, or meditate.

Grounding assists in the alignment process by supporting the foundation of one's whole self and field. In order to weather storms and ascend toward the light, we must be deeply rooted in the Earth. Energetically, I feel that grounding improves the overall relaxation of the mind and body, communication between the subtle bodies, the balance of the right and left hemispheres of the brain, sleep, the stress response, and resilience.

Grounding is especially important for those of us in urban environments because of the increased density of thought forms, electrical currents, Wi-Fi, EMFs, as well as light, noise, and air pollution. Trauma survivors can tend to have dysregulated responses to stress, and grounding promotes a more harmonized stress response. In a balanced state, we are comfortably rooted into the Earth, all our chakras are open, and we feel connected to our heart. I find that those with higher baselines of anxiety tend to experience an up-and-out energy pattern that can be problematic. Therefore, balancing this pattern by encouraging the energy to go in and down can be useful.

RITUAL | Grounding

You may want to experiment with one of the aforementioned grounding essences or an essence of your choice.

Sit comfortably, quiet your mind, and close your eyes if that feels okay. If possible, have your feet flat on the floor. Take some deep, grounding breaths into your belly and into your root chakra, which is located right around your perineum. Allow the lower part of your body (your feet, legs, thighs, and hips) to relax with each exhalation. Feel yourself getting heavy and sinking into your seat. Allow a grounding cord (I like to envision a tree trunk) emanating from you lower back, going through your root chakra, and plunging all the way to the Earth's crystalline core. Feel the Earth energy coming up through your lower body, through your root, and through your feet, with every inhalation. Just notice how you feel in your body as you connect with the Earth. Stay and hang out here for a few minutes.

When you feel ready to come back, gently release the grounding cord back to the Earth, and allow your root chakra to come to a comfortable, neutral position. Slowly deepen your breath once again, bring your awareness back to your space, and open your eyes.

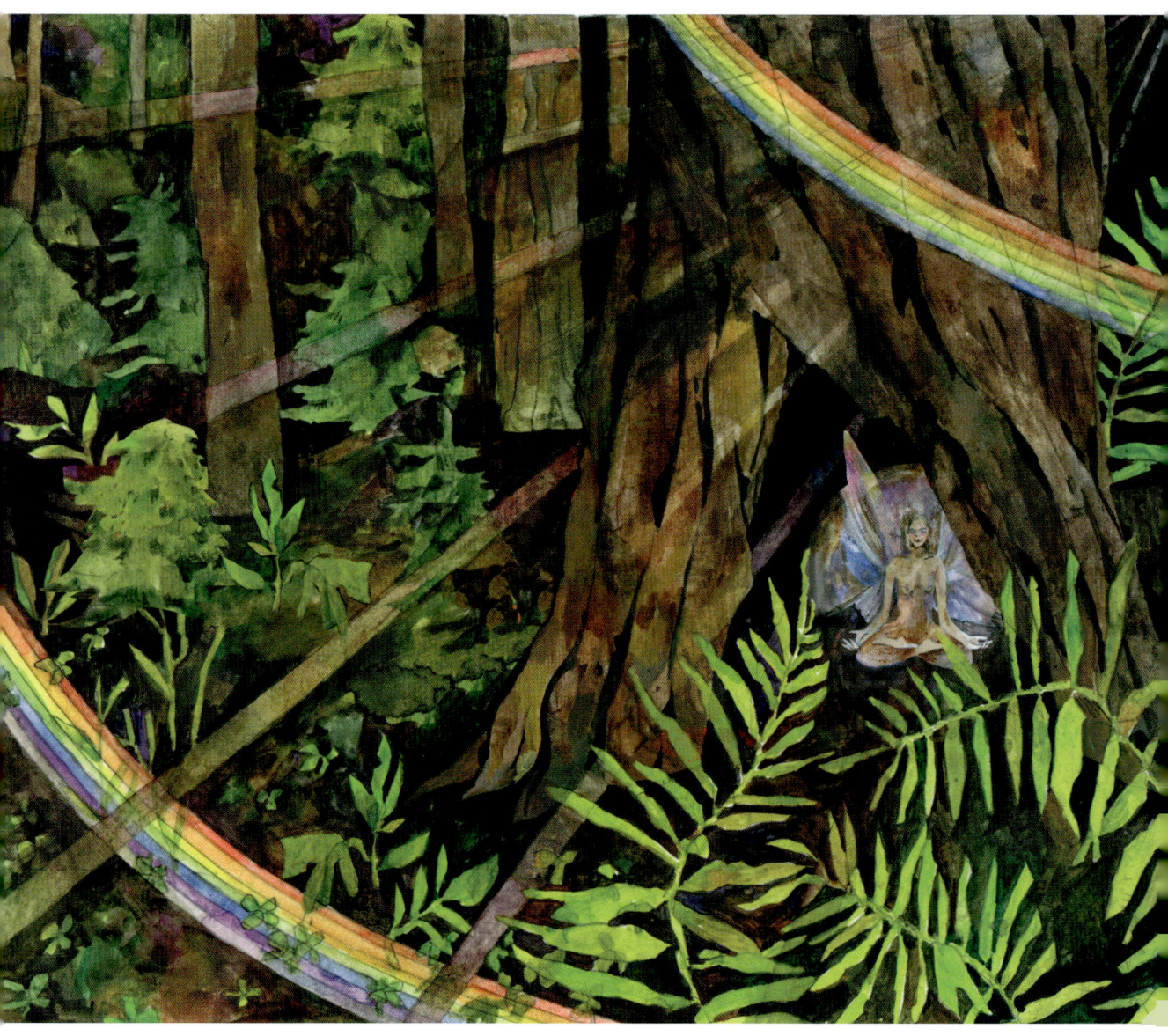

Some Protective Rituals

There are times when we need extra protection from the Universe. Some of us have been raised to believe the world is a dangerous place and that we are powerless within it. Even though we may sometimes feel helpless and alone, this is never the case. Hopefully, you will see the benefit of building a relationship with your angels, guides, and ancestors, who are here to support you and your work.

In addition to praying and grounding regularly, here are some of protective rituals I use:

- Ask that all you do be kept in the light, and to be shown what to do if a lesser light force intrudes.
- Visualize spheres of light around your body and auric field. Cobalt-blue for healing; white for purity; rose quartz for divine love; black tourmaline to repel negativity and toxicity.
- Imagine a shower of light bathing your auric field (an egg-shaped energetic membrane) and washing all the psychic debris off, then flowing back to the Earth.
- Take an actual bath and consider adding Epsom salts, sea salt, and sagebrush flower essence.
- Utilize stones or talismans by wearing them or placing them near you. Black tourmaline is excellent for grounding toxicity, and smoky quartz is good for repelling negativity.[12]
- Have a clearing practice after work, such as using a flower essence mist around yourself when you're done for the day.
- Take a flower essence, such as AE Soul Support, FES sagebrush, or DG Clearing.
- Regularly clear your home. Utilize palo santo, sage, cedar, incense, or any ethically sourced plant you like to burn responsibly. Energies may collect in closets and corners. This includes purging items you don't need. Ask yourself: What are you holding on to that may no longer be serving you?
- My friend and healer Eloise Christensen taught me to always ground the light you surround yourself with. Imagine tucking it under your feet like a blanket.

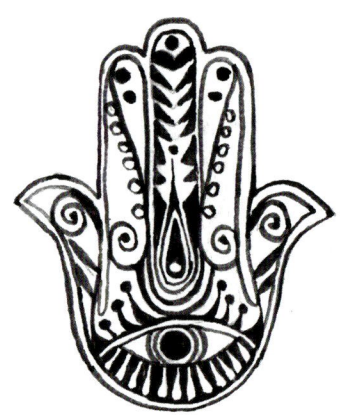

Working with Intention

In the last chapter, we discussed intention when making a flower essence. In terms of ritual work, working with intention is the process of bringing more consciousness to your healing practices. A common misconception about spirituality is that it is separate from your daily life. But, in truth, how you do one thing is how you do all things. This includes what you choose to think, believe, say, and do. Everything contains a vibration which creates resonance, which then affects the material or physical plane.

Working with intention isn't difficult, but it does require practice. You need to invest some energy in those areas of your life where previously you were just going through the motions. If you make a regular practice of setting intentions, you will gain the ability to shift the energetics around your intentions. Working with intention is foundational to manifestation, a more advanced skill that will be covered in a future text.

If you are offering a healing practice, your intention becomes a big part of the vibrational signature of your offering, whether it be physical or subtle energetic (vibrational) medicine. Be creative, work with art, nature, or whatever inspires you! Energy follows intention. Wherever you place your intentions, the energy will show up there. Here are some flower essences to help you bring more intentionality into your practices.

Flower Essences for Working with Intention

DG red passionflower—for new beginnings; for setting intentions; for overcoming hatred, anger, greed, fears of lack of resolutions to overcome the lower self.

DG briar rose—to enhance spiritual practice for those who are developing a spiritual discipline; helps maintain connection to the heart when one seeks to discipline mind and body; for busy and dedicated personalities who suppress their feelings.

DG lovage—for moving into the world with a sense of safety and joy; confidence in taking action.

FES blackberry—positive qualities: competent manifestation in the world; clearly directed forces of will, intentional and decisive action; and patterns of imbalance: inability to translate goals and ideals into concrete action or viable activities; procrastination.

FES star tulip—positive qualities: sensitive and receptive attunement; serene soul disposition; inner listening to others and to higher worlds, especially in dreams and meditation; patterns of imbalance: inability to cultivate quiet inner presence, lack of attunement or soul insight, unable to meditate or pray.

FES tansy—positive qualities: decisive and goal-oriented, purposeful in action, self-directed mastery and achievement; and patterns of imbalance: lethargy, procrastination, inability to take straightforward action, habits which undermine or subvert real abilities and talents.

"Write it down. Spelling is a spell."
—Erykah Badu

Abundance and Privilege

Sometimes the intentions of our rituals are centered around a desired outcome. And much of this time, our desires are linked to abundance. Abundance need not always be tied to the material, but to the actualization of a desired state or experience, such as wanting to connect with love. Let's explore this intersection of desire and abundance, and how it is impacted by our privilege.

What is true abundance? And what is a result of one's privilege? I came across this query on Instagram a few years ago, and it gave me much to ponder. How much of our privilege is part of what we actually manifest? What is our karmic destiny and where do we have the power to make different choices that shift our fate? These are places where I sit in inquiry instead of arriving at simple, tidy answers. I do believe that we create our own realities. Even in the depths of my own despair, which was serious depression, I believed that I had the power to turn things around for myself, and I did. However, none of my journey—from a rudderless boat in a stormy sea back to shore—was separate from the gifts with which I have been blessed. I had the financial support of my family and my partner to go to school, train, and build a new career. I had the ability to access mental health care. I had the unconditional support of friends and teachers. It would be tone deaf and inappropriate for me to say to a client who can barely pay the rent and take care of her children to "just manifest a different outcome." It is a very ableist assumption that someone can simply will themselves out of a survival state, regardless of circumstance. There are times when we have the opportunity to will things into form and action, and other times when we are asked to wait, or watch, or to be patient. I am continually amazed at the resilience and grace that arises when we come into alignment to trust ourselves and surrender to the divine plan.

Not everyone has the same access to manifesting and generating abundance on the physical plane. Remember, the dominant culture is a system that reinforces white, cisgender privilege and oppresses all who don't identify with these demarcations. Yes, anything is possible. And, forces such as institutionalized racism and bigotry are limiting and opposing forces that don't make the playing field level—in the physical plane anyway. The dreams and desires of the soul, the alchemy of spirit, communion with nature and the divine—these are domains beyond the physical, and the patriarchy has no dominion over them. This would explain why indigenous traditions and any practices involving self-empowerment are threatening to the establishment. In the spirit world, all things are truly possible.

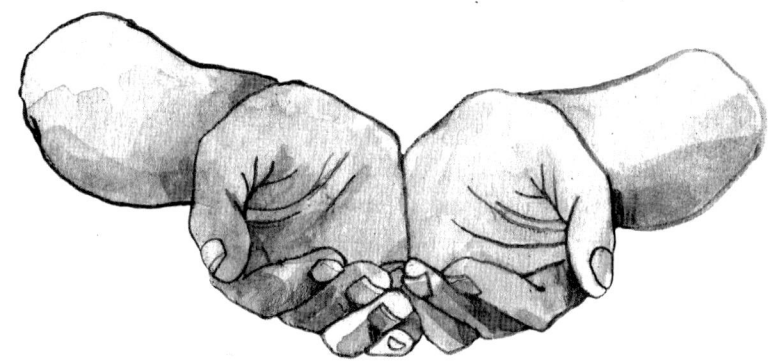

What do you seek? Being human means being attached to needs and desires. (If your practice is working toward nonstriving and desiring nothing, then good for you! Personally, I'm not there yet.) Our current identification with prosperity is inherently tied to the duality of the patriarchy. It's okay to want to generate your own abundance, as long as it's for the higher good. What you need to remember is that you cannot fear lack and attract abundance at the same time, a classic paradox of the egoic masculine. A lack statement is something like: "I don't have enough" or "If only I could get this, then I could feel that." On the other hand, statements such as "I am grateful for what I have, and I would like . . ." or "The Universe is providing me with exactly what I need, and I would like to invite in . . ." attract abundance instead of magnetizing your thoughts and beliefs to more of what you don't believe you have. The beliefs that you give the most energy to will be what you successfully attract into your reality. You are living in a Universe that is made up entirely of energy. You yourself are energy. The Universe is infinitely abundant, and therefore it can never "run out" of energy.

We have so much more opportunity to be supporting each other, despite the capitalist cultural conditioning to be in competition with one another. Personally, I've grappled with jealousy, believing that when another woman was championed, I was somewhat diminished. This may have its roots in evolutionary biology, but perhaps the survival consciousness of "more for you equals less for me" is not rooted in reality. What someone else is creating doesn't take away from what you're creating; it can only support it. Competition is rooted in the patriarchy. Collaboration is rooted in the divine feminine. We are here to create. Creation and abundance are infinite. One person's awesomeness can't negate someone else's.

THERE IS INFINITE SPACE FOR EVERYONE TO BE AWESOME

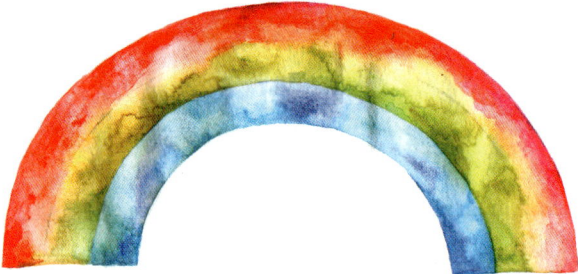

If you're only focused on generating a certain kind of abundance, you're limiting other kinds of abundance that can come your way. Viewed through the lens of scarcity, one would assume that only so much creation or abundance is possible. Leave room for the unknown and never assume you know better than what the Universe can provide for you. It's also a lot more fun to consciously make space for unexpected gifts.

Because we operate within a disproportionately egoic masculine culture, there is a lot of fear floating around. We are also highly sensitive beings. Therefore, our relationship to abundance needs to be evaluated, because what we are culturally glorifying becomes the subjective goals of the masses. If our society defines abundance from a place of ego, we, too, are subject to reinforcing fear (for example, I need to be rich and look young to get love), instead of abundance for the higher good (I need to generate wealth so I can do what I love and fulfill my purpose on Earth).

There are many beings who exemplify impressive mastery in the material, third-dimensional realm, but perhaps it's time to celebrate the unique brightness of every individual. Imagine if our society celebrated emotional integration as much as we did finances, if we honored teachers as much as celebrities. Many times, the idea of who's "special" and "brilliant" is also tied to the egoic masculine, and what meets the current cultural standards of beauty and ableism. Recognizing that's the dominant model, you can choose to participate or not, and begin to see all beings as vessels of unique and brilliant light.

We've run out of time to be thinking small and scarce. Dreaming abundance into being must be for ourselves *and within* the context of the greater good for all. Ask yourself: Is this desire compassionate to my soul? To others? The world? May we all magnify abundance and succeed together, in whatever ways we are called to bring our light into the world.

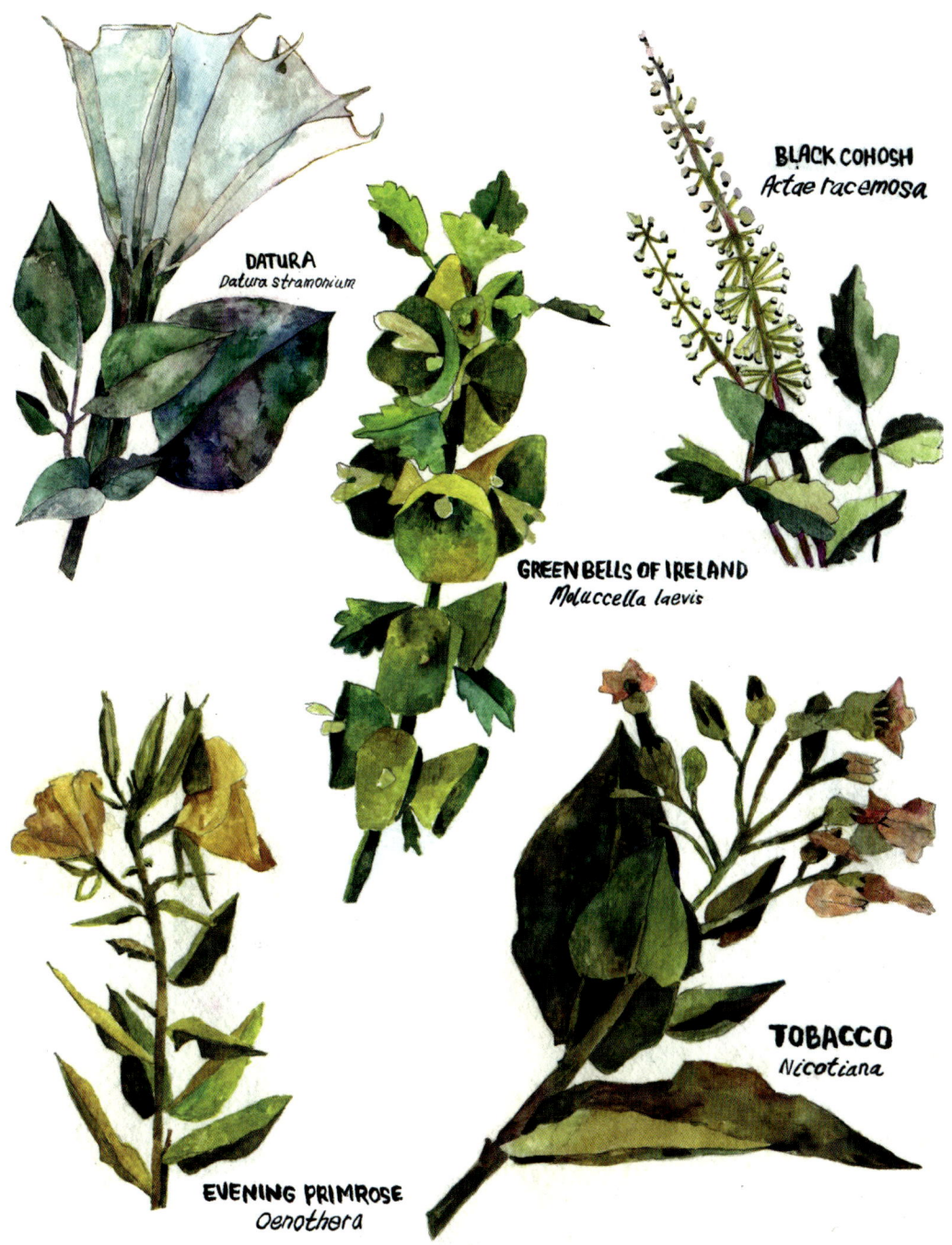

The Moon, Medicine, and Ritual

What does the moon have to do with flower essences and ritual? As we discussed in an earlier chapter, the moon represents a time before the dominant culture came into power. While the moon has no gender, it is a metaphor for the divine feminine and a symbol for the creative, the intuitive, the unconscious, and the shadow. Before the Gregorian calendar came into use in the sixteenth century, many cycles of time were measured on a lunar basis, as are the Islamic, Chinese, and Jewish calendars today. All ancient agriculture was organized around lunar and astrological transits, which is one of the basic practices of biodynamic farming today. Many of us feel a fascination with the moon, and I feel it beckons us back to a different consciousness, where much healing potential awaits.

In the following sections, I will offer some of the wisdom shared with me by a few of my fellow practitioners. I love getting to hear about how other herbalists and healers have the same fascination with the moon as I do, and how they honor the moon in their practices.

 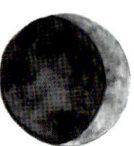 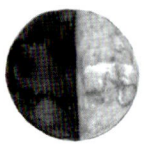 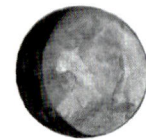 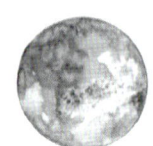

Making a Moonlight Essence

If you are curious about incorporating the energies of the moon in your work, making a moonlight essence is a beautiful ritual to employ.

Here, flower essence practitioner, producer, and teacher David Dalton shares his method for making a moonlight flower essence.

Moonlight Flower Essence, by David Dalton

The year 1995 was a turning point for me in my flower essence work. Before that year, I had religiously followed the Bach method of making essences—three hours in the rising sun. In 1995, everything changed. My garden began to manifest odd flowering patterns—different colors and shapes; some plants bloomed out of season or for a second time. My inner guidance spiked that year, and I began a project to make essences within the lunar cycles over the spring, summer, and fall.

Starting in the early spring, I would pick the flowers from six or seven plants and place them in separate jars with pure water, and store them in a corner of the garden until the full moon. At the full moon, I would uncap each jar, place it in the moonlight on a stone in the center of the garden, and witness an unusual display of light and sound. Tiny filaments of light would cascade into the jar and a chant (a different one for each jar) would appear in my mind first and then escape from my throat. By November, I had collected thirty-six of these essences and, although I felt unusual energy coming from each of them, I was uncertain how to use them. I stored them in a safe place with a preservative and then forgot about them.

In December that same year, a voice awakened me from sleep and instructed me to bring all the essences out under the moon (it was full then) for one hour. The next day, I had my first and only experience of automatic writing, and wrote out brief, somewhat metaphysical descriptions for each of the essences. These descriptions appear now on our website, deltagardens.com.

Ten years later, I was able to record the chants that accompanied the essences into form. Although the quality of the sounds and the essences are not precisely in the Bach tradition, they have a sweet and unusual presence and are used by many practitioners today.

David Dalton is a flower essence practitioner, producer, and teacher. He is the founder of Delta Gardens and the author of *Stars of the Meadow: Medicinal Herbs as Flower Essences*.

Shadow Work: The Dark Side of the Moon

We are all ascending, together. The de-evolution, disintegration, duality must be unified individually and collectively; there is no separation. How we heal ourselves impacts the field of others and the Earth. Jung defined the shadow as the part of the self that was not fully conscious, and therefore unintegrated. The shadow is usually responsible for lower vibratory states that we experience.

> *Shadow work is the path of the heart warrior.*
>
> CARL JUNG

Many ancient teachings remind us that the point of life is not to perpetually chase after pleasurable feeling states, a purgatory of the third dimension. However, we are designed to feel higher, lighter vibrational states: joy, peace, love. The more shadow you clear, the more light you let in. The higher you desire to ascend, the deeper in the dirt you must dig to balance the duality. As Jane would frequently remind me in our work together, "No muck, no lotus," which are the words of Zen Buddhist Thich Nhat Hanh.

With the encroachment of technology and the general sense that everything must be done immediately, young people especially are vulnerable to the egoic perception that all is instantly attainable, even enlightenment. This spiritual egotism occludes the purpose of shadow work. The shadow works on the schedule of the moon. Everything has a time. There are voids. There are unknowns.

How do you work with the shadow? Everything you do to support yourself assists you in holding space for duality and tolerating the discomfort of the shadow. The shadow is the ego personified, so all egoic identification will show up somewhere in the shadow. The conflicts that arise between the ego (mind) and the heart (soul) commonly present in the physical, mental, or emotional body. Since the progression of the shadow moves from unconscious internal projection to unconscious external projection, the implications for shadow work are paramount.[*]

---

[*] From interpersonal discord to political corruption, it's easy to see how many of the world's issues arise from a lack of awareness about one's shadow. Shadow projection is the original blame game. If someone doesn't feel like taking responsibility for their own stuff (emotions, thoughts, actions, memories, stories, relationships), they will likely project it onto a vulnerable person or group. The "family projection process" is the intergenerational means by which this happens in family systems.

It is also possible to unconsciously take on the shadow of others and the collective. Empaths need to be particularly careful to avoid doing this. While it is a valiant impulse to try to help an individual or a group by processing their shadow for them, it prompts a sort of psychic codependence that can turn the murky wateriness of your work into a sea of volatile waves. In short, unconscious shadow work can be dangerous and disorienting.

There's a reason temporary episodes of insanity are sometimes referred to as "lunacy." Perhaps the wise ones before us recognized the gifts within the negative aspects of the moon, such as the unhinged qualities it can evoke in us. There are times of the month and year when the veils are thinned, and access to the shadow and the invisible realms are enhanced. Shadow work can present as instability, and there is healing available to us in allowing the disintegration to happen in order to consciously reintegrate.

Working with your shadow requires a certain level of mastery, and it's a good idea to have a guide, someone who has tested and swam in the waters themselves. Jennifer Patterson of Corpus Ritual will share some ways she works with the shadow in a bit.

> *The Moon stays bright when it doesn't avoid the night.*
>
> RUMI

Working with Lower Vibratory States

Shadow work is going to be uncomfortable, there's really no way around it. Can we lean into this discomfort? I have found that when we are in pain, it is helpful to ground our energy. There is insight on the other side of this discomfort. Just as we do in Focusing, can we name what is coming up and allow it to be there? Combining an intention around the state you are exploring with the earlier grounding exercise is a powerful ritual you can cultivate on your own. Two of the most frequently presenting lower vibratory states I encounter are depression and anxiety. How can ritual assist you in working with lower vibratory states?

One of the places flower essences really excel is in working intentionally with thoughts and belief systems. Interestingly, while antidepressants are one of the most heavily prescribed class of pharmaceuticals, it's been shown that the placebo effect, or believing that something will work, is just as—and in some cases, more effective—than actual medication.[13] This points to the power of affirmation and prayer.

Let's say you are really struggling with anxiety. For instance, you feel a pervasive sense of dread and your mind races before bed. Choose a flower essence to work with, either on your own, or from the following list of my most-used essences for working with lower vibratory states. Again, practice the grounding ritual. And this time, when you are noticing how it feels to connect with the Earth's energy, begin to notice any felt sensations in your body. See if it's okay to name them. Feel into these sensations a little bit; it could be uncomfortable. Now, see if it feels okay to allow them to be here. If this feels like too much, simply open your eyes and reorient yourself in your space. See if you can safely work toward acknowledging the felt discomfort and breathe into it. Notice what happens when you do this.

My Most-Used Essences for Working with Lower Vibratory States

This could be an exhaustive list, and rather than give you every single one, I'm offering the ones I call on most often. As your flower essence work deepens, you, too, will gravitate toward certain plants. It can be helpful to notate which ones you find yourself reaching for most frequently.

DG angelica—provides assistance in sealing the energy field that is challenged or compromised from growth, processing, or developmental movement; a wonderful essence to assist anyone going through periods of rapid change.

FES borage—positive qualities: ebullient heart forces, buoyant courage and optimism; and patterns of imbalance: heavy-heartedness or grief, lack of confidence in facing difficult circumstances, depressive behavior.

BE Mimulus—"the bravery flower," from fear of the world to trust in the world; "[develops] the Soul's potential for courage and trust."[14] For confidence to face daily challenges and fears; for those prone to phobic personality; positive qualities: courage and confidence to face life's challenges, radiant light that shines outward to the world; and patterns of imbalance: over-exaggerated concern for daily life events, extreme apprehension of new thresholds of experience.

BE pine—"the self-acceptance flower," from self-negation to self-respect; "[develops] the Soul's potential for self-acceptance";[15] positive qualities: self-acceptance, self-forgiveness, freedom to move forward despite past mistakes; and patterns of imbalance:

melancholic obsession with past events, overemphasis on guilt or self-blame, paralysis due to excessive self-criticism.

AE tundra rose—indications: hopelessness, lack of inspiration and motivation, overwhelmed by the responsibilities one has taken on; and healing qualities: restores hope, courage, and inspiration to those who have much to offer but are close to giving up; strengthens the ability to bring a more robust expression of joy and enthusiasm to the fulfillment of one's responsibilities.

DG pearl/lilac—elixir of hope, expansion, and upliftment; take one drop per dosage for best results; one feels the purest essence of love and support.

Beware of the Bypass

Usually, when we come up against discomfort, there's a tendency to resist or contract to avoid feeling pain. Bypassing is a natural response to pain because we have been taught to avoid painful emotions and lower vibratory states, believing they are bad and dangerous. It requires practice to discern when to lean into discomfort and when to move the energy in another way. Being aware of how we bypass helps us cultivate this discernment in our shadow work.

Bypassing arises when the work of confronting the ego or the shadow seems too overwhelming. It's a defense mechanism, a way to numb out, to avoid feeling the negative emotions that accompany therapeutic work. When there is deep-seated resistance to something, the ego can fool us into bypassing. So, what is seemingly beneficial is actually keeping us in a place of unconsciousness. It can be a fine line sometimes. Virtually anything can function as a bypass. A few examples of bypassing include overwork, staying in a toxic relationship, ostensibly following a belief system, teaching but not integrating therapeutic work on a deeper level, or using a particular teaching or practice to avoid feeling uncomfortable. Bypassing always involves some kind of unconscious projection of the shadow.

Among the ways to keep from bypassing are to honor where we are in our process every day, to stay in witness of whatever is coming up, to honor our whole selves, and to remember that ascending is not easy or painless. I've found lemon balm to be helpful in therapeutic work where resisting or bypassing can occur, as it helps to relax and create a safe container to go deeper. Working with someone to keep us accountable is also a good option. The ego can trick us into believing that anything painful should be avoided. But in the wise words of healer Mary O'Malley, *What's in the Way Is the Way*.[16]

> *People that meditate exactly the right number of minutes, eat exactly the right food, do all the things perfectly, can also be caught in the chain of gold, in the chain of righteousness and ritual. That is not liberation.*
>
> RAM DASS

EXERCISE | A Ritual in Surrender

Bypassing is a type of resistance. When we are in resistance, we always have the option to move into acceptance. The practice of surrendering is one way of letting go of what doesn't serve us. When I think of plants that encourage surrender, Bach's pine essence is what first comes to mind, as it is known as the self-acceptance flower. The act of surrendering may need to be an ongoing exercise. This ritual is best done regularly and works well if you have access to fresh water such as an ocean or stream.

Sit quietly and ground your energy by breathing into your belly and root. Call all your energy into your being and come into presence. Allow yourself to connect with something that is causing you trouble and hold it in your awareness. Notice any physical sensations that arise when you do this, paying special attention to any sensations of contraction, tension, or resistance. Without getting hooked into the story or judgment about the sensation, see if it's possible to just sit and be with it. Next, see if it's possible to transfer into your hands that physical sensation that is causing you pain. You can visualize it moving like an orb, surrounded in rose quartz light. Allow your breath to help you move the energy into your hands. Then place your hands on the ground or in water. I like to bow my head and breathe for a few moments. Be sure to say thank you for this teaching and to the Earth.

I myself struggle with intrusive thoughts, a form of hypervigilance I continue to heal. To me, they feel like a rigid swirl of energy in my head. Intrusive thoughts are an opportunity for me to surrender, and sometimes I need to do this practice throughout the day, when I don't have access to water or much time to sit and reflect. In this case, I simply name the intrusive thought as soon as I'm able to catch it. I notice how it feels in my body, then I invoke surrendering, and say, "Thank you, I release you."

Poison Medicine and Shadow Work

It's easy to separate our natural world into a good/bad binary, for example, good plants and bad plants such as weeds and invasive species. A lot of the plants that hold poisonous properties also have a special affinity to the shadow and the in-between places, or liminal realms. Jennifer Patterson is an herbalist and breath work practitioner who explores the often-misunderstood application of poisonous plants in her practice. Here, she shares her method of making a *Datura* flower essence along with a breath work exercise.

EXERCISE | *Datura* Flower Essence and Breath Work, by Jennifer Patterson

To make an essence, first make sure you are able to accurately identify the plant. If the plant grows plentifully, and is not on any at-risk lists, you can start by sitting with the plant. By building up your relationship to the plant's energy, after some time you can ask the plant for its consent in harvesting a few blooms or portions of the plant to sit in a bowl of water under both the sun and the moon. We want that moon energy, that darkness, to infuse our essence too. But be cautious. Janet Kent, of Medicine County Herbs writes: "[I]f, when asking a plant permission to harvest, you have never heard 'no' then you aren't listening. That voice that always says 'yes' is your own." If you don't want to take any plant parts, or as a way to work with rare and at-risk plants, you can also bring two jars with you—one full of water and one empty. Pour the water over the plant, catching the water in the other jar, over and over, until your intuition guides you to stop.

Blooming at night with the sweetest single drop of nectar the morning after, Datura is a remedy for holding us between the poles of dark and light, a reminder that they are mirrors. As void medicine, it helps guide us through the emotional and energetic threshold and freefall of releasing what is no longer serving us. To allow for a death, or an ending, invites space for the new to bloom. The death that is needed can be parts of ourselves that require release, old narratives that bind us to the past, relationships and dynamics that don't serve our growth, and more. It invites real, sustaining connection and aliveness that exists under all the wounding and old harmful patterns. It's bold and fiery: medicine of the underworld. It supports welcoming the open palm instead of believing that clutching tightly is the only way through.

AFFIRMATIONS FOR RITUAL WORK

I believe in the wisdom in the void. I welcome the death of the old to make room for new relationships and dynamics with myself and others.

BREATHING PRACTICE FOR CALLING THE PARTS BACK

The breathing practice is intended to be a way for us to reconnect to our bodies to help create a container for intentional ritual work. For many of us whose bodies have lived through violence, sometimes bringing attention to the breath, and our bodies, can be triggering. Before beginning the practice, set up a comfortable and supportive space. Open by telling yourself that you consent to this practice, that this practice is in service to you, and may help reframe any fears that might be showing up. Repeat as needed.

Sit or lie on a yoga mat, floor, or bed. Set a timer for five minutes, building up to ten minutes over a few days' practice. When you feel ready, I invite you to close your eyes. If at any point you need to reorient yourself in the room, feel free to open them before shutting them again when you feel steady. Begin with a long, slow inhale, about five counts, through your mouth, feeling your belly and chest expand. Slowly exhale for about five counts through the mouth, quickly bringing the inhale back in for another five counts. A few minutes into the breathing, see if you can notice your toes, your calves, your knees, your hips, and so on, scanning up your body. You don't have to figure anything out or linger in any place for too long. When you get to your heart ask yourself:

What parts of me have been cast off or rejected?

What kinds of support do I need to call them back?

What do these parts need from me in order to feel safe to return and integrate?

Continue this breath until the timer goes off. Give yourself one more minute of any kind of slower breath. Send yourself, and those brave parts that spoke up, your gratitude and your love.

If the questions feel difficult at first, keep trying. Sometimes these parts of ourselves just need to know we are dedicated to them and that we are working to invite them home. After the breathing practice, take a few drops of your essence, in support of integrating what you just learned. If you'd like to also take a few minutes to write or draw, this creative practice can help you retain some of the wisdom you've found.

For all of us striving for "well," "healed," and/or "whole," may we remember our healing (active and ongoing) is all tangled up with each and every other person. We cannot be "well" when the world beyond us is very unwell. We cannot be "well" when we have deemed parts of ourselves, or others, as bad or wrong. It doesn't mean that we should act out of these wounded places, or let them run the show, in fact it's quite the opposite. By tending to these places, with love and care, we can give these lonely parts, often in deep isolation and pain, what they need: witness and acceptance.

Jennifer Patterson is a grief worker, writer, and speaker who uses plants, breath, and words to explore surivorhood, body(ies), and healing. She is a queer and trans-affirming, trauma-experienced herbalist and breathwork facilitator and editor of *Queering Sexual Violence: Radical Voices from Within the Anti-Violence Movement*.

Menstruation and the Moon

The practice of syncing one's menstrual cycle with the moon is called lunaception. At the time of writing this, women's health care has become increasingly under attack, and being in touch with one's natural rhythms is more important than ever. The following offering by somatic psychotherapist Deborah Bagg highlights a way to honor and connect with one's menstrual cycle, a sacred rhythm unambiguously linked to the moon. This topic has garnered much popularity in the last few years. And if the idea of talking about periods makes you cringe, maybe step back and observe why. Why is it that a normal human function—responsible for human life itself, that provides us with much information about the state of our physical, emotional, and spiritual self—makes you uncomfortable? Can you see the power available when you call back this part of the human experience, this part of yourself?

Honoring and Connecting with Your Menstrual Cycle, by Deborah Bagg

A huge part of working with myself on an emotional level during my moon cycle has been using flower essences. I recommend them to my clients in my somatic psychotherapy practice. Flower essences can be a supportive tool to integrate through each particular phase. I have noticed a trend in each phase and have provided flower essences that I feel are most often beneficial in supporting the process. The Bach essences chosen are to support the positive potential and alignment of each honored phase. (These are all Bach healing herbs.)

FOUR PHASES OF THE MENSES MOON CYCLE

1. New Moon Phase—The Menstrual Phase:
   A time of deep listening, introversion, slowing down, and self-care.

   Cerato: If you are feeling uncertainty and disconnection from yourself, needing external validation and approval, take Cerato to connect to your intuition for guidance and self-trust.

   Cherry plum: When you're feeling out of control, overwhelmed, perhaps having suppressed what needs to be felt or heard, take cherry plum to restore tranquility, release extreme emotions, and express yourself calmly.

   Olive: If you are feeling depleted, exhausted in body, mind, and spirit, olive helps to restore and renew vitality.

2. Waxing Moon Phase—Preovulation:
   A time of relief, coming out of retreat and starting to integrate yourself back into the world.

   Larch: When you need a boost of confidence to step forward into your life, take larch to foster self-unfolding and self-esteem.

   Scleranthus: This flower could be helpful to support decision-making that got illuminated during your menses. Using the wisdom gleaned in new moon, you make choices to support your vision.

3. Full Moon Phase—Ovulation:
   A time of productivity, social activities, and engaging in life and the world around you.

   Water violet: When you're feeling guarded, wanting to withdraw, and distancing yourself from others, take water violet to support connection and relatability.

   Mimulus: When you need to connect with your bravery and courageous self, take *Mimulus* to work with the fears that hold you back from actualizing what you want in life.

4. **Waning Moon Phase—Premenstrual:**
   A time of transition, when you may feel aggravated and intense, when daily life doesn't accommodate your preparation into your menstrual retreat.

   Impatiens: When you're feeling inner restlessness, irritation, and annoyance, take Impatiens to calm yourself, increase patience, and slow down.

   Walnut: When you are feeling supersensitive, vulnerable, and needing healthy boundaries, take walnut to support you in this transition and change. It's a powerful remedy of protection.

I invite you to notice, and engage with, your personal moon cycle. Some people bleed with the new moon, while others may bleed with the full moon. Some cycles are longer, some shorter. Being mindful of your personal cycle can offer you an opportunity to build a deep and empowering relationship within yourself. Track your cycle's rhythm and flow, and become curious and intimate about what your body is communicating to you. Let the changing nature of your body be the guide to your mental, emotional, and spiritual growth.

Deborah Bagg, LMHC, is a somatic psychotherapist, yoga teacher, birth doula, and flower essence therapist. She is the owner of Jupiter Yoga & Healing Arts and co-owner of Spirit Shop.

EXERCISE: Planting a Moon Garden

Creating altars or sacred spaces outdoors can be another place for ritual work. While I can't have a moon garden in the city, I can have a few lunar plants in my windowsill to catch the moonlight.

Not all flowers bloom in the sunlight. Some plants prefer the darkness, opening to the night. Moon plants can be cultivated in any terrain. Many night bloomers are also very fragrant. I consider all plants medicinal to some degree; however, some of the moon garden plants may be more therapeutic than others. These can also be plants that you use for making your own flower essences. Or, if you like to make dried sticks of herbs to burn, you can use the plants from your moon garden, such as mugwort.

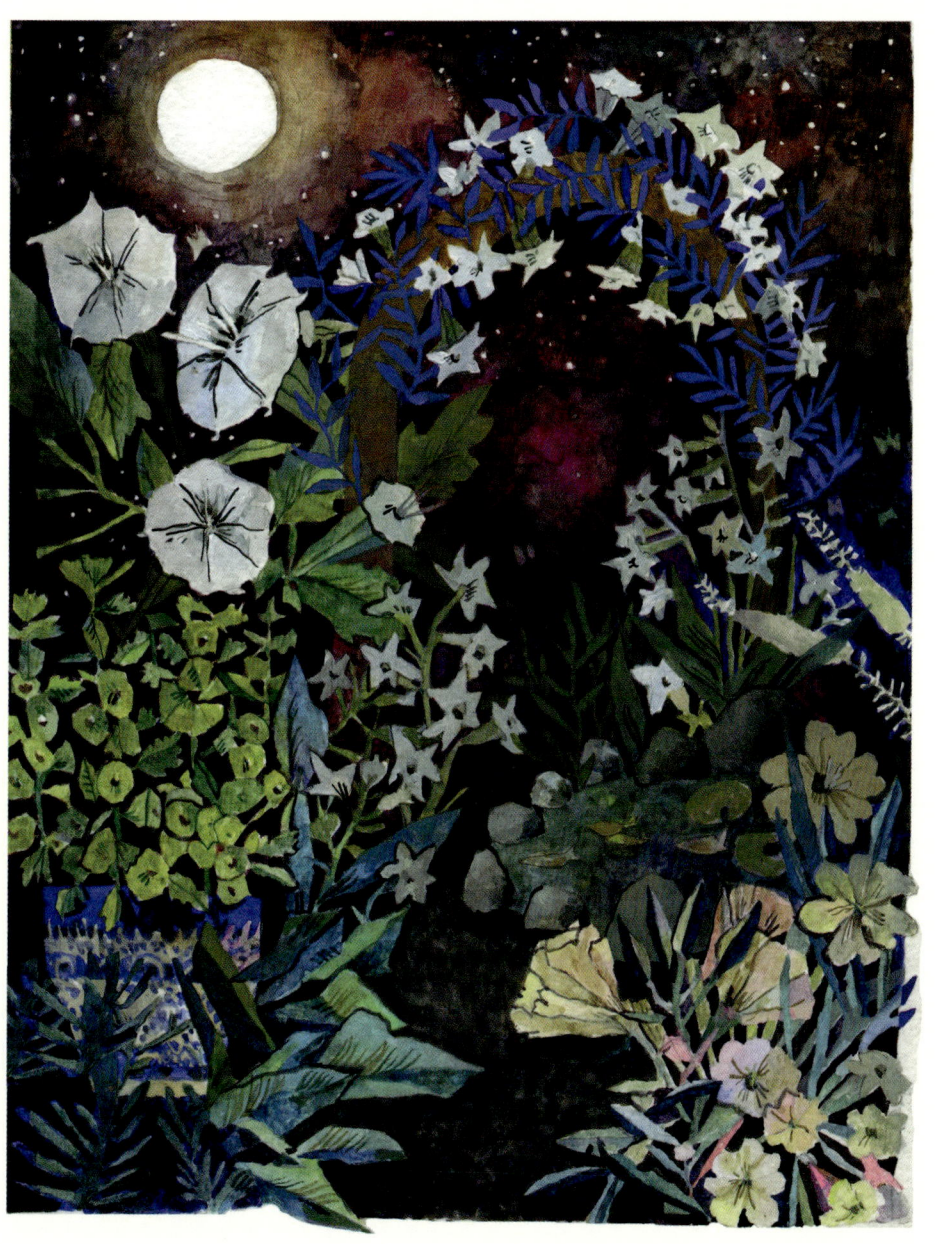

You can see the lunar signature of mugwort by observing the underside of the leaf, which is silver. The Latin name for it is Artemisia vulgaris; Artemis, *if you remember, was the Greek goddess of the moon! Plants with light and white blooms work best, as well as gray and silvery leaves.*

Here are some perfect moon garden plants:

- *Moonflower: emits a citrusy scent and is in the morning glory family*

- *Nicotiana: a sacred native tobacco plant that gives off its fragrance after sunset*

- *White angel's trumpet: has a beautiful downward-facing bloom*

- *Datura: a poisonous plant known for its psychedelic properties*

- *Mugwort: used for releasing energy and dream work*

- *Lamb's ear: a hearty plant that features wooly, soft, silvery leaves*

- *Silver sage: has aromatic silver-gray leaves and grows well in desert conditions*

- *Night-blooming jasmine: a divine-smelling shrub*

- *Lily of the valley: features small bell-shaped flowers that emit a beautiful scent*

- *Gardenia: has large white blooms that also have a heady scent*

Honoring Death and Loss

Many societies, both in antiquity and presently, hold very different relationships to the rituals surrounding death, loss, grief, and memorialization than our dominant culture. Celebrating *Día de los Muertos*, or the Day of the Dead, has extended to many parts of the world. Samhain is a Celtic pagan holiday honoring the dead. In ancient Egypt, death was seen as an initiation—not the end of a journey, but the beginning of one. Because the collective is currently identified at the level of ego, there is a tremendous fear of death, as the ego can only rule the physical domain. Therefore, death equals loss of control and ultimate annihilation. This means that we

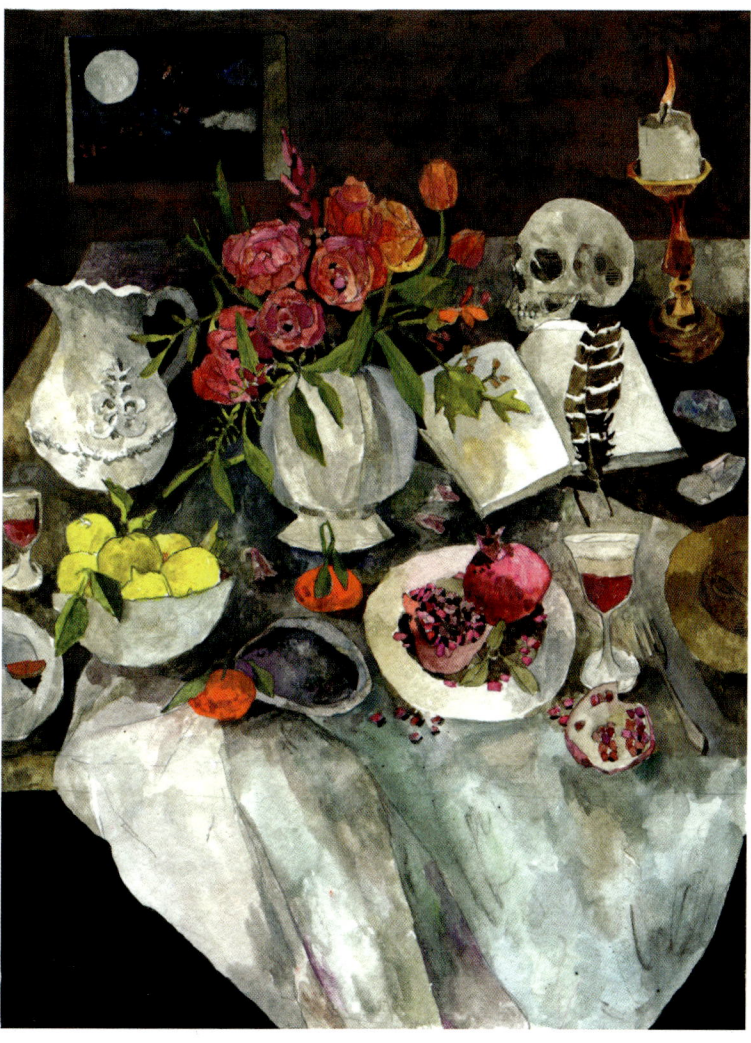

are very much oriented away from accepting death as a natural part of life and treat it like a disease.

Grieving can extend to any kind of loss: the end of a relationship, the end of an era, a surgery, illness, a move, a job change, a loss of physical ability, a miscarriage or abortion, and so on. Grief is something Western cultures have a conflicted relationship with; thus, there are places where we could use more ritual and support to help us navigate through death* and loss. For example, military personnel return home with post-traumatic stress disorder (PTSD) due to the extreme loss they must inflict and endure. Unfortunately, adequate resources don't exist for this population to heal and adjust back into civilian life. According to the *Diagnostic and Statistical Manual of Mental Disorders*, grief experienced for longer than two months following a loss is considered clinical depression.[17] It can feel invalidating when there is no ritual or, at the very least, a cultural acknowledgment that it's okay to have an emotional response to death and loss.

Grief can be individual or collective. It can be very clearly situational or more abstract. For many sensitive beings, the devastation to the Earth and her inhabitants can bring tremendous grief. Indigenous groups include cumulative and historical trauma, which can be understood as "collective and compounding emotional and psychic wounding over time, both over the life span and across generations" in their conceptualization of trauma and resultant grief.[18] It seems that here, too, a more inclusive and holistic approach to working with death and loss are in order.

How do we support others during a profound loss? This is something most of us haven't been taught how to do from a very conscious place. In the beginning of my work as a counselor, it was extremely difficult for me to hold space for people in pain because I hadn't yet learned to manage my boundaries and energy; I felt others' pain very acutely. Then, I would instinctively want to alleviate their pain instead of allowing them to process it on their own. Later on, through watching how trusted practitioners and elders held space for grief and loss, I learned that sometimes there are no words or deeds to help, but that just your presence is a gift. If you can hold an unconditionally supportive container for others to say or do whatever they need to, that is being of high service.

---

* In *The American Way of Death Revisited*, Jessica Mitford confronts the largely unregulated, capitalist nature of the funeral business in America. Perhaps unsurprisingly, the arbitrary rules, lack of choice, and obligations foisted upon the grieving party are a reflection of the conflicted relationship Americans hold toward death.

Days honoring birth, accomplishment, and union are important to celebrate. Death and the ending of things should likewise be memorialized. Endings can be doorways, thresholds to other realities and consciousnesses. Many of us subconsciously hold on to dates of loss because they inherently cry out for expression. In the pagan tradition, Samhain, October 31 and November 1 are the days when the veils between the living and the dead are at their thinnest, making connection with energies that have passed on more accessible. Someone who discusses this subject with great wisdom and heartedness is Chelsea Granger, who has also graced the pages of this book with her magical artwork. I recommend connecting with her work to learn more.

When my brother passed in 2007, I was confused because I didn't know how to mourn him. We weren't very close, so I struggled to find ways to honor his life and received mixed messages about honoring his death. People assumed that because he was my brother, I shouldn't be too upset, or that after one year I should be "over it." It took me a while to find ways to remember and memorialize him. Now I talk to him when I go running, because he was a runner. Sometimes I light a candle and say a prayer, or I tell a story about him. Whenever I travel somewhere new, I always ask him to come along to experience it with me. Although we didn't have much of a relationship when he was alive, his spirit will never be forgotten. He was very much a part of the creation of this book, and I couldn't have done it without his unconditional support. It might sound strange, but I actually feel closer to him now than before he died.

Sometimes not having a ritual to commemorate a death or loss can create a stagnation. For example, grief can get stuck in the lungs, negatively impact the sexual organs if there was some kind of sexual or reproductive trauma, weaken the heart, or present as a general state of malaise. When we stifle the cries of loss, they congregate in the throat chakra and can lead to imbalance and infection. The stories and emotional attachment surrounding death and loss can get tuned to a perpetual bandwidth, leaving us unable to move forward.

Some questions to consider: How can a loss inspire greater connection for you? Is there some creative expression that wants to emerge from your experience?

Some other ways to honor death and loss are:

- lighting a candle and saying a prayer
- writing a letter and offering it up
- traveling to places and making offerings for a person or an experience

- having an altar or place with pictures and objects
- making a calming herbal tea with herbs such as rose, hawthorn, lemon balm, or chamomile
- planting a tree or garden
- connecting with nature (sometimes supportive signs will present themselves)
- holding a remembrance circle or vigil

We must give ourselves permission to grieve and mourn, in whatever ways we feel necessary; even if there is no model for it, we can invent one. We should feel supported to grieve any loss that causes us pain—it shouldn't have to be "big" to be valid, such as losing a loved one as opposed to losing an animal. We should feel supported to process grief whenever it arises, outside of linear time and space. The moon encourages us not to fear the dark or the doorways. Everything that falls will rise again. The veils that separate us are not so impenetrable. Love never dies. Energy never dies, it merely morphs into something else.

Loss and Grief Flower Essences

FES Post-Trauma Stabilizer—a blend of arnica, bleeding heart, Echinacea, glassy hyacinth, green cross gentian, fireweed, five-flower formula, and essential oils of lavender, yarrow, and hyssop; for loss or disruption of any kind that creates bewilderment, numbness, or shock in the body-soul complex.

BE rock rose—"the liberation flower," from panic to heroic courage; develops the Soul's potential for courage and steadfastness; transcendent courage when facing adversity.

BE honeysuckle—letting go of the past, coming into the here and now so that life can go on after death or loss; for acceptance of circumstances.

DG stinging nettle—for releasing pain and grief related to partings and endings; for those who are often in conflict with others; for healing deep hurt from abandonment.

DG catalpa—promotes the release of old and deep pain that has caused difficulty in the lung-heart area; for processing unresolved grief from childhood or past lives.

DG small white aster—for those who know they will pass on; heals shock, self-pity, and grief; strengthens certainty in relationship to the Divine; helps the soul prepare to travel.

FES angel's trumpet—positive qualities: spiritual surrender at death or at times of deep transformation; opening the soul to the spiritual world; and patterns of imbalance: fear of death, resistance to letting go of material life and crossing the spiritual threshold; denial of the reality of the spiritual world or the soul's need for change.

FES or DG borage—uplifting and renewing the heart with courage; heart balm for grief.

FES yerba santa—internalized sadness due to past trauma, melancholy; deeply internalized pain stored in the heart and chest.

FES Grief Relief—pink yarrow, bleeding heart, love-lies-bleeding, California wild rose, borage, forget-me-not, and explorer's gentian; solace and insight in times of sorrow and searching.

Dream Work

Dream work can be a potent self-discovery tool. Everyone dreams, although some people recall their dreams more than others. Dreamtime is rich terrain for archetypal exploration. The ancients heeded the messages and advice in their dreams, as we would from a trusted source. From an energetic perspective, every night the astral body literally disconnects from the physical body and floats around in the astral plane. There, our psyches can mingle with influences and energies within the collective. It is no wonder that children sometimes fear sleep; it is actually quite wild to think about the journeys we go on each night!

On a physical level, our body is undergoing much regeneration while we're asleep. Our cells regenerate, our brain cleanses itself, each of our organs and bodily systems are encouraged to reset themselves—all this happens during sleep. It's not possible for many of these deeply restorative actions to occur while we're awake. (An exception would be deeply meditative states, which mimic and can even enhance many of the restorative and rejuvenative processes.) Sleep is of profound importance for our health and well-being. In our modern world, sleeping and dreaming have been cast aside in place of overwork and productivity. Theta waves are the frequency of the brain as we are falling asleep, and are associated with flashes of insight, vivid creativity, and deep relaxation. Delta waves are the slowest waves emitted by our brains in between dreaming (and also meditation); they are necessary for much of the regenerative functions of our system.

Therapeutically, dream work can be a way in when no solutions or signs present themselves in waking life. Lucid dreaming is the practice of co-creating the landscapes of your dreams in collaboration with your subconscious. This can be particularly useful in repetitive dreams, where your subconscious is attempting to tell you something. One is not limited to time or space in dream work. It is possible to give yourself a signal to realize you are dreaming, and control the dream however you desire. Resolving conflict, exploring a time or place, reconnecting with someone, experiencing pleasure, flying—all are possible in our dreams and can be deeply reparative on many levels. I've had the opportunity to resolve deeply and long-held conflicts that wouldn't be possible in waking life. Skeletons in my closet present themselves, and we can reach a place of appreciation and forgiveness. I have no doubt that these dream encounters are clearing karma in the physical world.

Dream journaling is a good option, either for deeper exploration of the psyche or for persistent issues that feel buried in the subconscious. If you have trouble recalling your dreams, try meditating before bed and setting an intention so that you will remember your dream upon waking. Dream dictionaries can be useful, but are highly subjective. I'm fond the general Jungian dream analysis theory, wherein all parts of the dream represent parts of ourselves. What does a particular symbol or theme in your dream mean to you? How does it feel to see that symbol as part of yourself? According to Liz Migliorelli of Sister Spinster, dream journaling works well when it is part of an ongoing practice. "It's like taking herbs; if you don't take the herbs frequently, they don't work in the body. If you don't show up to writing the dreams down, you won't be able to develop a deep relationship to your dream vocabulary."[19]

I have had success with taking a flower essence for dream work before bed, setting an intention, giving myself a signal if I'm engaged in lucid dreaming, and writing down what I've dreamed as soon as I wake up. I will then choose a way to integrate the meaning of the dream by writing or drawing about it. Bringing the insights from your dreams into waking life ensures to your subconscious that you got the message.

Bombarded by nightmares or disturbing dreams? We all go through periods when we're trying to work things out, and so much healing is happening while we're sleeping. Many variables may contribute to this phenomenon: medication, disease, substance use or withdrawal, PTSD, or acute shock of any kind. If you suffer from night terrors, these can sometimes be a form of astral intrusion, and being mindful of protection and psychic protection can be helpful.

Bedtime Rituals

- Practice healthy sleep hygiene: create a dark and quiet room with little to no electronics; limit screens before bed or download a filter that offsets the blue light of your screens.
- Take an Epsom salt bath; the salt pulls out impurities and eases muscle tension.
- Place a warm compress over your eyes, with a couple drops of lavender or chamomile essential oil on the inside of the cloth (not making contact with eyes) for an added relaxing effect.
- Get a white noise machine or download nature sounds to help your brain turn off.
- Journal: What were you grateful for today? Or write down all those thoughts that might be keeping you up.
- Meditate: Try taking one of the flower essences below that calls to you, and sit quietly for a few minutes. See if you can just notice what's coming up and allow your body to prepare to sleep. Ask for permission to connect with the spirit of whatever flower you have chosen, and ask for its help in whatever ways you need support.

Dream Work Flower Essences

BR angelica—provides protection from the spiritual worlds and the help of loving forces from on high; "angelic protection," especially when one crosses the threshold to the "other side," for example, in situations such as death or passing away, dreams, meditation, operations, or serious illnesses, when the mortal body is less bound to the Earth.

BE white chestnut—for restless, fitful sleep due to anxious feelings or repetitive mental chatter.

FES star tulip—for greater receptivity and awareness of dream symbolism and dream recall; more awareness of subtle realms.

FES chaparral—for disturbed or chaotic dreams; release of trauma, sometimes through catharsis; cleansing of the psyche.

FES forget-me-not—to facilitate communication and connection with spirit guides or departed souls in dreams and sleep.

FES mugwort—for awareness across the threshold; greater activity and consciousness in dreams; integration of dream life and psychic awareness with ordinary reality.

AE Guardian—a blend of covelite, devil's club, round-leaf orchid, stone circle, white violet, and yarrow; helps you create a powerful force field of protection in your aura; it invokes positive, harmonious energies that help you claim your energetic space, maintain your grounding, and feel the protection of strong, healthy boundaries.

DG Soul Dreams (moonlight mugwort)—brings forward deeply held dreams, desires, and fears for releasing or embracing; permits functional levels of manifestation to bring in blocked desires; helps us reawaken "wanting" in alignment with our soul.

DG St. John's wort—provides a sealing and strengthening to the energy field that is weakened from shock, burnout, or from an expanded or escapist nature; protects from dreamtime imbalances; the sealing action of this essence occurs from within the energy field in the area where the field connects to the belly.

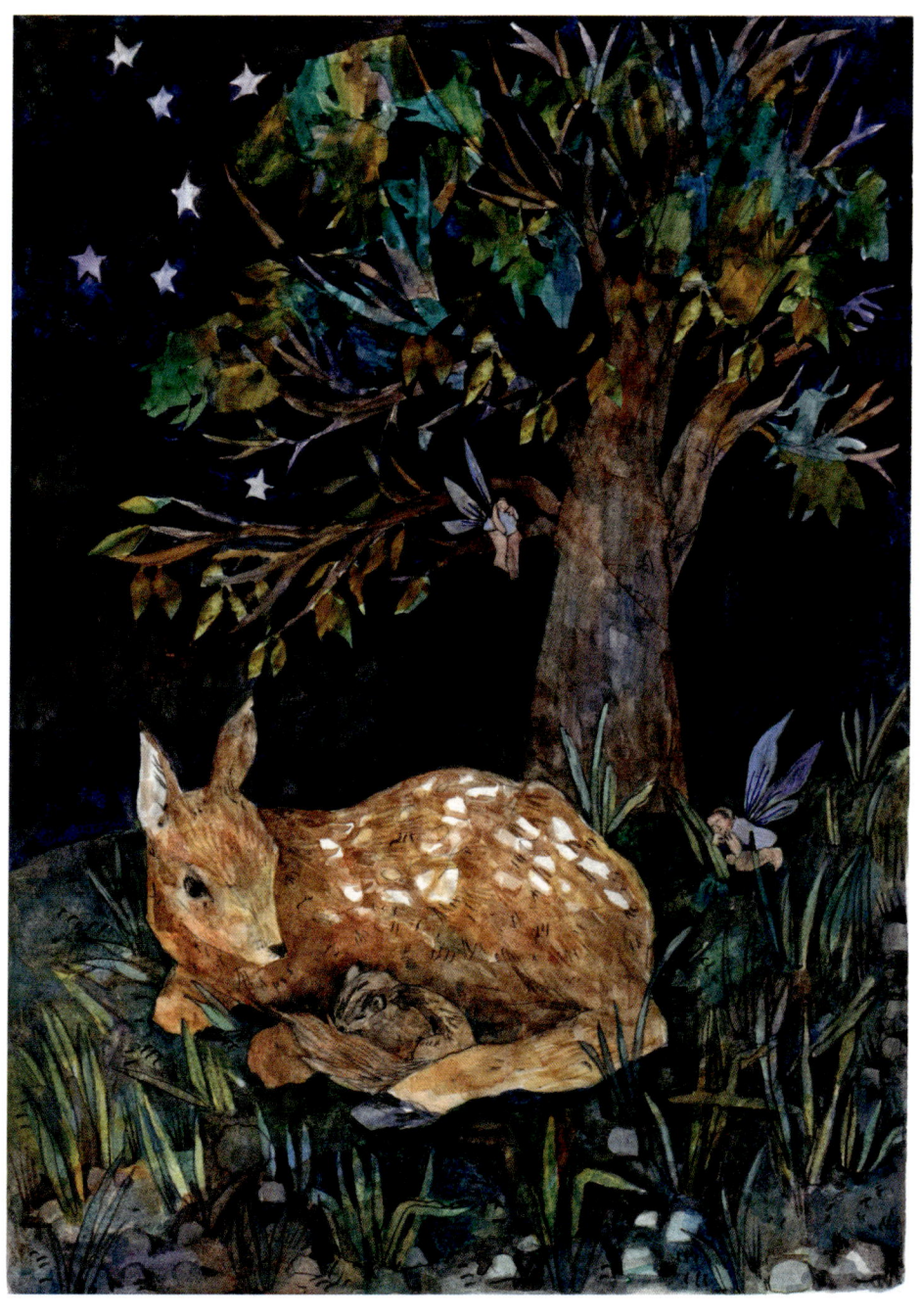

Heart Medicine Rituals

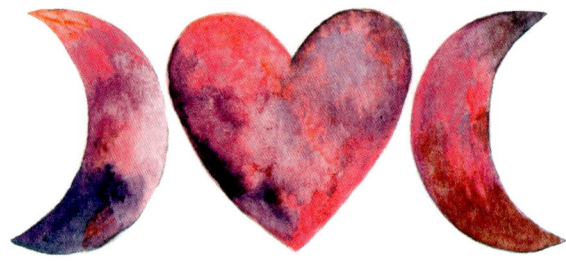

*The heart chakra is the central integrating chamber
of the chakra system. Through the healing power of love, all things
eventually find their way to connection and wholeness.*

ANODEA JUDITH

The greatest lesson I have learned so far is to exist within my heart. This is a lifelong practice for me, because like many, I was not taught to inhabit my heart space. On a physical level, the general collective is not doing so well in our hearts. This is evidenced by the stark reality that heart disease is the leading cause of death worldwide.[20] This high incidence of disease points to a deeper situation of the heart, but in order to be open to the possibility that more profound heart healing is necessary and possible, we must open our minds to a more metaphysical or energetic interpretation of what the heart is and what it does. Ancestrally, the heart held a much higher evolutionary significance, and as our consciousness split, we moved from inhabiting our hearts to glorifying our minds. Perhaps this disconnect can illuminate some clues for us to consider to reclaim more balance within our hearts, ourselves, and our world.

Vibrationally, the heart contains the strongest electromagnetic field of any organ in the body.* Transference of heart energy can occur in close proximity with another human or animal; and if you apply the theories of quantum entanglement and wave

---

* The electrical field as measured in an electrocardiogram (ECG) is about sixty times greater in amplitude than the brain waves recorded in an electroencephalogram (EEG). Heart Math Institute, 2010.

function collapse, transference of heart energy can resonate beyond space or time.[21] Plants and the elements, too, can have a positive entrainment effect on the heart, reiterating the interconnectedness of all life and the organic balance nature engenders. In both traditional Chinese and Tibetan medicines, the heart *is the mind*. In TCM, grief is stored in the lungs and closely related to the heart. The Hopi defined harmony as one's heartbeat in resonance with others and the Earth.

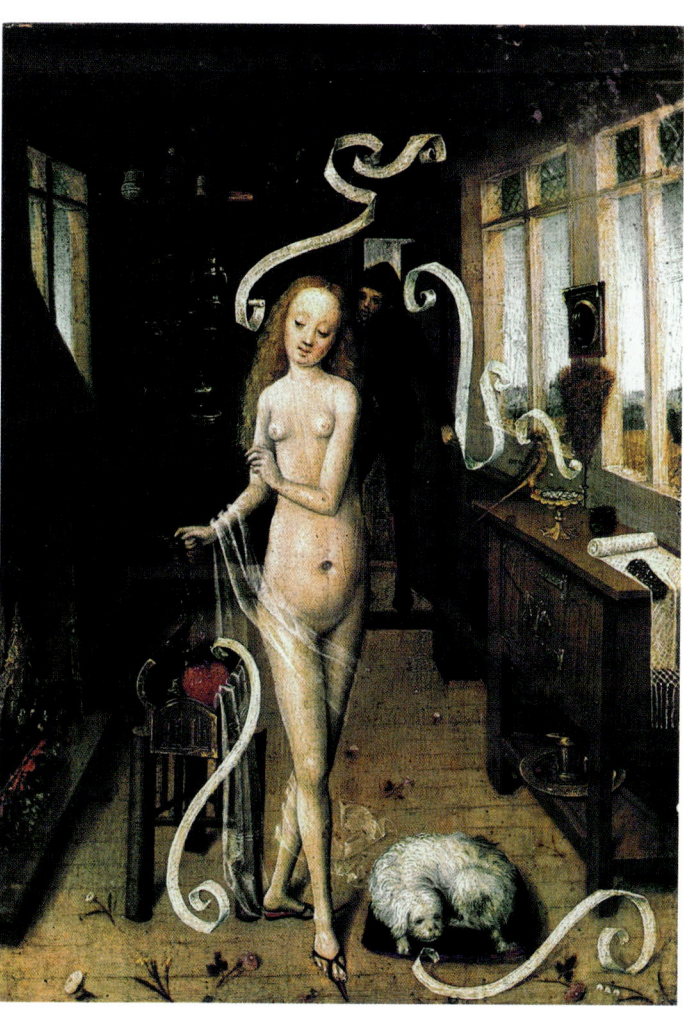

THE LOVE SPELL, lower Rhenish painter (fifteenth century).

Our liberation is tied to the heart. The cost of liberation is unique to every person and is cosmically linked to each of us. The price of liberation varies for each individual, but we are given choices: in what we think, what we feel, what we believe, how we want to be. The inability to see choice is the unconsciousness of the fear-based toxic masculine that seeks to keep us disconnected and disempowered.

Our liberation depends largely on our ability to love unconditionally. Unconditional love means loving without circumstance or codependence. This can take different forms, from exiting a toxic relationship to taking more care of yourself. And it doesn't stop there. If you want to get really free, you have to love yourself no matter what, and love all beings no matter what. Tall order? Yes. Impossible? No! While humans are conditioned to be in separation, plants (and animals) hold only unconditional love for all life. There are people on this Earth who radiate unconditional love, and when you are in their company, your heart is completely relaxed and open.

For instance, my heart feels completely free when I am with people and animals who love me unconditionally. My heart also feels free in this way when I am in nature. Can you think of anyone who loves you unconditionally? Or perhaps it's easier to think of an animal or pet? What if you loved yourself and everyone like that? What if you loved all your uncomfortable parts, illnesses, and neuroses like that?

Jane was my guide back to myself, back into my heart. I carry her expert guidance in the work I do with my clients when we collaborate on our therapeutic intentions: how we decide the client will be best served by our time together. Regardless of what is decided upon, or how it evolves, the heart is always guiding the process. We will always work to connect with the heart center, whether we're working with anxiety or depression, childhood trauma, life transition, or serious physical illness.

Talking is a helpful part of the therapeutic process; however, bringing the awareness into the body and heart is where deeper healing occurs. Most people benefit from getting out of their mental bodies (the intellectual, masculine mind) and into their hearts. As much as we've been conditioned to believe that we can heal from an intellectual place, it's simply not possible. You must feel what you want to heal. The heart is the cosmic gateway to this healing process.

Unconditional love is the ultimate dissolver and healer. The field of unconditional love is the optimal state of balance and unity, in which maximum potential is activated. Unconditional love can exist anywhere in one's being and field, and is activated most notably in the heart. We are learning much interesting new data on the heart and healing. The heart sends far more signals to the brain than the brain sends to the heart.[22]

In order for us to survive and thrive in an increasingly volatile world, we must integrate the mental (masculine), emotional (feminine), and meet in the heart (soul consciousness). Using the mind and the heart together to make decisions is the embodied process of discernment. Others call engaging the heart and mind together simply the "heart-mind."

As infants, we were completely open and heart-centered. As we sustained traumas and the conditioning of life, our hearts shut down. In Focusing, I encounter much armoring around the heart. Most of us are walking around with multiple walls around our hearts that we erected in order to feel safe. For instance, if you feel a lot of negative projection from your family, you may notice a lot of armoring around the back of the heart, which can manifest in a tightness of breath and upper back pain.

When you inhabit your heart, and it is in balance, your heart center is open on all sides and relaxed. When the heart is open, we can generally enjoy the following with greater ease:

- equally giving and receiving love
- connecting authentically with others
- existing within and experiencing states of appreciation, compassion, gratitude, and resilience
- experiencing states of bliss and wonder
- feeling safe, loved, and unconditionally supported
- the ability to move through obstacles and challenges with your higher self
- the sense of infinite potentials
- enhanced connection with present time
- enhanced ability to forgive and love unconditionally

Some ways into greater heart healing include:
- limiting excess (this includes negative thoughts)
- adequate, uninterrupted sleep
- proper diet and exercise
- meditation, especially a self-compassion or loving awareness practice

- breath work (the heart responds well to regulating via the breath)
- any practice that encourages theta waves (deep sleep and meditation, floating in a sensory deprivation tank, gong or singing bowl bath,[23] intentional resting near running water)
- being in nature (connecting to the heartbeat of the Earth)
- working with an essential oil such as rose, which has a special affinity for the heart
- connecting with supportive people
- connecting with animals in a loving and caring way[24]
- working with a practitioner who has a heart-based philosophy and practice
- volunteering or being of service to others
- working with flower essences such as rose, hawthorn, and borage

---

EXERCISE | Making a Rose Essence and Heart Breathing Exercise

---

There are a few plants whose application is almost universal, and the rose is one such flower. Roses hold the frequency of unconditional love and have an affinity for the heart chakra. This ritual works best with either a wild growing or organically cultivated rose; it can be any species within the Rosa *genus. Some of the lower vibratory states that can be addressed with rose include grief, loss, heartbreak, depression, and panic.*

This ritual is very simple. You're going to combine the process for making your own medicine (page 98) with the heart breathing exercise that follows. The heart breathing can be done while the flowers are in the water, working their magic. The heart energy you engage during the medicine-making process will become part of the energetic signature of your flower essence. After you bottle it and make the dosage bottle, take a few drops and see what you notice around your heart. Be sure to notate your findings. You now have a rose flower essence for your apothecary whenever you or someone else needs it.

HEART BREATHING

After you have placed the flowers in the bowl with the water, sit comfortably on the ground, if possible. Close your eyes or set your gaze low. Place both hands over your heart and begin to breathe into the heart space. Visualize the rose you are working with. Notice how the breath moves in and out of the heart—not forcing the air, just allowing it to move. See if you can sense into how the heart is feeling—in the front, in the back, all sides. Be sure to breathe into the back of the heart space. Notice how the heart feels when you place your awareness on it. See if it's okay to allow whatever is arising, witnessing without judgment.

After a few minutes, begin to bring the heart back into a neutral position. Thank your heart and the spirit of rose for sharing with you. Feel your body making contact with the Earth, deepen the breath, and slowly open your eyes.

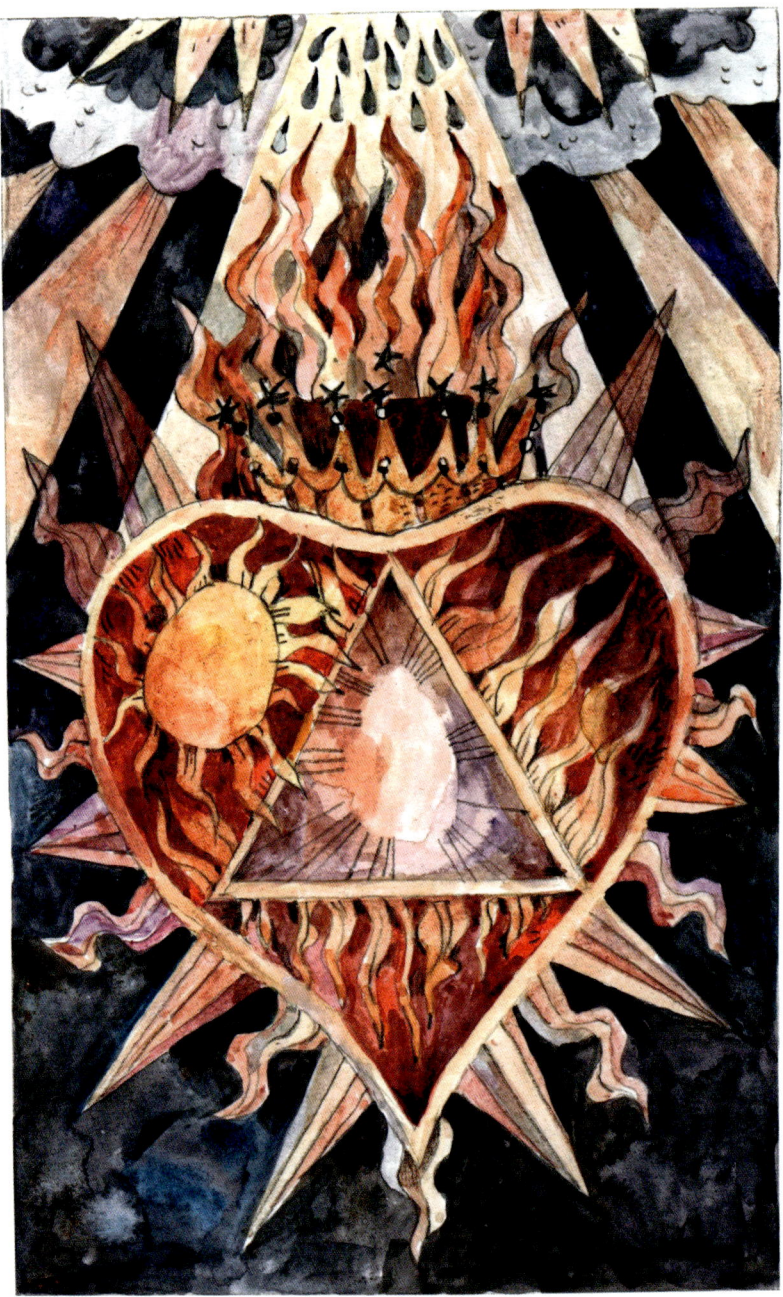

Tend and Befriend: Circling Together

The paradigm shift that is currently underway is happening in large part because people are waking up in their hearts—which feels like an encouraging sign for the future. We are wired for both pessimism and connection in times of stress. Though we have been largely conditioned to pull ourselves up by our own bootstraps and deny our needs, this is not the natural way. Women, in particular, possess special relational capacities that lend themselves to nurturing in groups in times of conflict. The phrase "tend and befriend" was coined by psychologist Shelley Taylor, with five of her colleagues, during their time at UCLA. She and her cohorts found that women actually excel at protecting and nurturing their kin in times of stress, while men tend to adhere to the fight-or-flight response, which triggers a different cascade of stress hormones in the system. Tending and befriending builds the attachment process in relationships and groups.[25]

As we move out of the time of separation, we are encouraged to reconnect to our true social natures. Women have always gathered in supportive circles: in red tents, in covens, around the moon. The yearning for community is a real desire for many of my clients, and for me. Whenever I work with groups, I'm continually blown away when I see the healing potential of those who intentionally gather together. The alchemy that arises in supportive circles cannot be reproduced—it is truly transformational. (**If you have the opportunity, I highly recommend making a flower essence with a group with a shared intention.**) Outside of a clinical setting, connecting with supportive people in times of need is healing on more levels than we are aware of. For instance, regardless of any negative attachment style we may have grown up with, our tend-and-befriend aptitudes repair the deleterious effects of even the most abusive early relationships. They teach us to trust, connect intimately, and open our hearts to greater healing.

When we factor in the role of healing justice in our work, tend and befriend takes on a new meaning. We are absolutely biologically attuned to heal the deep duality and oppression within ourselves and the collective. Healing and evolving together is the new paradigm we are entering. I hope you will consider how to make healing justice a priority in your personal and professional practice. I have listed more resources on page 207 for further study. Here are some essences to assist you on your way.

Healing Justice Flower Essence Allies

There are a number of herbalists and alternative healers who have been speaking on the subject of healing justice for quite some time, and I am grateful for their leadership and inspiration. These essences are wonderful to use in process groups or healing circles that center on antiracism and anti-oppression work. Some flower allies to assist you as you dig deeper into this rich and rewarding terrain are:

DG lemon balm—a wonderful essence for when you are immersed in deep work, to keep calm and carry on.

DG valerian—for any resistance to change, to be able to take in and assimilate new information.

FES quaking grass—"harmonious community consciousness," letting go of personal attachments in social groups.

FES lupine—seeing beyond the level of self, seeing self as part of the whole.

FES or DG Echinacea—integration of those parts of the self that may have been repressed.

FES or DG borage—to support the heart and offer courage.

BE water lily—for humility and wisdom in communication, to heal the perceived separation we feel from others based on race, class, or gender.

FES pink yarrow—for emotional vulnerability, assists in discerning what is your responsibility to emotionally process.

Conclusion: Flower of Life Activation

When I gather in circle, both with my guides and with my community, I go deep into my heart to feel what is there. From this place, I know we are here to heal together, to come back into unity. This is happening as the Earth is taking herself back. All those practices that allow information to come into our fields, to honor the Earth and her inhabitants, to help us reconnect and remember what has been forgotten—these are potent counterbalances to duality because they can integrate human and divine, matter and spirit, as within so without. The rituals that were stolen from us, what we were forced to forget or hide: now is the time to renew them and bring them into the light. The act of reclaiming and creating ceremony—from our intuition and ancestries—is a righteous and empowering act of love and letting go.

There were times during the writing process of this book when I felt discouraged and doubted that I could contribute something that would be of any significant value to positive collective change. One day, I decided to sit in meditation with this fear and see what arose. I took a drop of FES's green rose essence and was transported to a circle of beings. When I looked closer, I could see they were all of those whom I am connected to in spirit, in this world and beyond. Each of us was engulfed in light, and some were merely orbs. Each of us held our right arm behind the next being's back, with our left arm to the sky. Each of us was holding a circle of light in our left hands. From an aerial view, these circles created a grid of larger circles, until it created a giant illuminated flower of life in the sky.

I was shown that this flower of life is being activated now, all over the world, by those who are shining their own unique light together as one. My prayer is this:

*May we circle together and embrace all the ways
we are inspired to live our dreams.*

*May our light guide the journey into a new age of sun
and moon exaltation, where all sentient beings
are free to live in the fullest expression of their souls,
in harmony together.*

So be it.

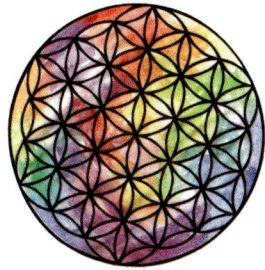

Acknowledgments

Loving thanks to all those who have believed in me and supported me on my journey to have the courage to write, especially my grandmother, Jane Stevens, and my mother for encouraging me as a child. My family, my original teachers. Jane Bell for saving and changing my life. My Universe partner, Will Welch, for loving me unconditionally and inspiring me to fully be myself every day.

My herbal teachers, Claudia Keel and Richard Mandelbaum, who are so expert and generous with their wisdom. My flower essence teachers: Patricia Kaminski, Richard Katz, and David Dalton, for their divine wisdom. My friends and colleagues, who offered me both practical and emotional counsel during my writing process: Deborah, Shenhav, Andrea, Alexa, Melissa, Bill, Nick, Karyn, Brooke, Michael, Phelicia, Crista, Raven, Aunt, Juliana, Virginia, Ana, Emily, Clare, Mark Anthony, Sinead, Liza, Aubrey, Natalia, Cate, Gretchen, Keely, Marie, Amanda, Jason, and Anna. To Hallie and Sherie, for supporting and encouraging me unconditionally.

Chelsea Granger, for being a genius and also one of the kindest souls ever. My amazing contributors who trusted me and my words and shared their work: Deborah Bagg, Jennifer Patterson, Lata Chettri-Kennedy, and David Dalton. My agent, Meg Thompson, who believed in me from the beginning, and whom I admire as both a business person and a human. My editor, Diana Ventimiglia, who was an angel and spiritual midwife to this project, and Jade Lascelles for all your help and kindness. To Sounds True, for being my dream publisher. To Maeve Carter, who generously shared wisdom with me gleaned from her extensive antiracism and social justice work. To Claire Howorth, Michelle Ruiz Andrews, Amanda Meigher, and *Vanity Fair* magazine: this abundance comes through thanks to you. To Kiri Fisher, my first mentor who totally shifted the trajectory of my life.

To all women who have silently endured trauma and survived. To all WOC, who inspire me to wake up. To all those with a commitment to protecting the plants, the animals, and the Earth. To my guides, angels, and ancestors, for their infinite guidance and protection. To Stuart, for lighting the way.

Appendix

CONTEMPORARY FLOWER ESSENCE PRACTITIONERS, RESEARCHERS, AND PRODUCERS

There are perhaps hundreds of flower essence producers in the world today, and this number will likely continue to rise. I will highlight a few whose essences I use in practice, and with whose work I trust. The Flower Essence Society and Delta Gardens spend a number of years researching essences before offering them to the public. They are very thoughtful about the medicine they share. Many contemporary flower essence producers follow the rituals developed by Edward Bach. Others follow more indigenous practices connected to various ancestries. As you begin to experience the essences of various producers, you will notice that each one is different. Because we are dealing with vibrational medicine, the energetic qualities of each of the producers are unique to that practitioner. Some will resonate with you more than others.

Healing Herbs Bach Flower Essences: These are the essences created by Julian Barnard according to the careful preparation instructions of Dr. Edward Bach, who produced the original 38 Bach Healing Essences. This set is an excellent foundation for beginners and practitioners alike. Julian Barnard is considered the leading expert on the English flower essences. The Healing Herbs and Bach Center in Wallingford, United Kingdom, conducts clinical research and studies on the efficacy of flower essences. Julian is the author of several books, including *Bach Flower Remedies: Form and Function* and *The Bach Flower Remedies: The Essence Within*.

Flower Essence Services (FES): FES is directed by Richard Katz and Patricia Kaminski, who are married and professional partners. FES handcrafts flower essences and related herbal products at Terra Flora, their twenty-seven-acre cottage industry, garden, and wildlife sanctuary in Nevada City, California. FES was founded by Richard Katz in 1978 after he researched and taught extensively about the Bach flower essences, herbalism, and botany. The FES product line is dual certified USDA organic and Demeter-Biodynamic and includes flower essences, essential oils, and related herbal products in various modalities such as dropper bottles, mists, creams, and oils. FES also distributes the Healing Herbs original Bach flower remedies in North America.

Delta Gardens: Founded in the mid-1980s by David Dalton, Delta Gardens is located in Hampton Falls, New Hampshire. David has been making flower essences in New England research gardens and in natural habitats throughout the world for over thirty years. Since the beginning of his exploration of flower remedies, David has combined clinical thinking, intuition, and a strong relationship with nature to create an extensive collection of products that support emotional, mental, and physical health. David is especially interested in the applications of flower essences to physical issues and Lyme disease. He has a special appreciation for the role of the chakra system and the art of manifesting. Delta Gardens features a wide array of both individual flower essences and sets from all over the world, gem elixirs, mushroom essences, and a set of moonlight essences. Delta Gardens offers various practitioner trainings throughout the year. David is the author of *Stars of the Meadow*.

Alaskan Essences: A unique system of vibrational healing based on the co-creative relationship that exists between the plant, mineral, and elemental kingdoms. They offer flower, gem, and environmental essences; and combination formulas and sprays, including several for pets. Founder, Steve Johnson, is the author of The Essence of Healing and the "Living Book," Alaskan Essences' Online Repertory.

Woodland Essences: Created by herbalist, Ayurvedic consultant, and flower essence practitioner Kate Gilday in Cold Brook, New York, these essences have a sacred relationship to the woods. Kate offers sets of tree, shrub, and forest floor essences, as well as chakra blends and at-risk North American flower essences. Her herbal product line also contains many tincture blends and topical preparations that include her flower essences. She teaches at various locations in the Northeast throughout the year.

Green Tara Flower Essences: These are produced by Julia Graves, who brings her experience of herbalism, traditional European medicine, gestalt psychotherapy, and anthroposophic massage to her remedies. Her essences share a particular affinity for the feminine, and her line includes a large number of lily essences. She teaches all over the world and is the author of *The Language of Plants: A Guide to the Doctrine of Signatures*.

Bloesem Remedies: These are created by Bram Zaalberg in the Netherlands. Bram has been wildcrafting his essences since 1986. He feels his remedies "work at a very deep level and are best suited for people who are willing to work on a more profound and spiritual part of their being." Bloesem Remedies offers standard sets, combinations, and a New Times set, intended to support individuals and the collective through our evolution.

Where to Find Flower Essences Online

Alaskan Essences Inc.
alaskanessences.com/collections/flower-essences/flower-essence-practitioner-kit

Bloesem Remedies Nederland
luminesce.ca/bloesem-remedies-netherland-flower-essences-of-the-netherlands.html

Delta Gardens
deltagardens.com/pages/flower-essence-sets

Flower Essence Services
store.fesflowers.com

Green Tara Flower Essences
lilycircle.com/flower-essences/

Healingherbs Ltd.
healingherbsdirect.co.uk*

Perelandra Ltd.
perelandra-ltd.com/Essences-Sets-C17.aspx

Woodland Essence
woodlandessence.com/Essences2.htm

---

* I strongly suggest ordering Bach essences exclusively from Healingherbs Ltd. or Flower Essence Services.

Notes

PREFACE

1. "A Quote from Epistle to the Hebrews," Jewish Women's Archive, accessed February 22, 2019, jwa.org/media/quote-from-epistle-to-hebrews.

CHAPTER 1: INTRODUCTION AND MY JOURNEY

1. Richard Gerber, *Vibrational Medicine: The #1 Handbook of Subtle-Energy Therapies*, 3rd ed. (Rochester, VT: Bear & Company, 2001), 252–253.
2. "It's Official—Spending Time Outside Is Good For You," *Science Daily*, accessed October 1, 2018, sciencedaily.com/releases/2018/07/180706102842.htm.
3. Cara Page, "Reflections from Detroit: Transforming Wellness & Wholeness," Incite! (blog), Aug 5, 2010, incite-national.org/2010/08/05/reflections-from-detroit-transforming-wellness-wholeness/.

CHAPTER 2: COMING INTO COSMIC BALANCE

1. Anne Kent, *Rush, Moon, Moon* (New York: Random House, 1976).
2. Jules Cashford, *The Moon: Myth and Image* (New York: Four Walls Eight Windows, 2002).
3. Teresa N. Washington, *Our Mothers, Our Powers, Our Texts: Manifestations of Àjé in Africana Literature* (Bloomington: Indiana University Press, 2005), 63.
4. Silvia Federici, *Caliban and the Witch: Woman, the Body and Primitive Accumulation* (New York: Autonomedia, 2004).
5. Sam Kriss, "The Patriarchy Hates the Moon," *The Atlantic*, April 5, 2017, theatlantic.com/science/archive/2017/04/why-the-patriarchy-hates-the-moon/521853/.
6. Bessel van der Kolk, *The Body Keeps the Score: Brain, Mind, and Body in the Healing of Trauma* (New York: Penguin Books, 2015).
7. C. Gilligan, interview by L. Granek (video recording), Psychology's Feminist Voices Oral History and Online Archive Project, September 15, 2009, New York, NY.
8. Deepak Chopra and Menas Kafatos, "What is Cosmic Consciousness?" The Chopra Center, chopra.com/articles/what-is-cosmic-consciousness. "Quantum theory has

reached the point where the source of all matter and energy is a vacuum, a nothingness that contains all the possibilities of everything that has ever existed or could exist. These possibilities then emerge as probabilities before 'collapsing' into localized quanta, manifesting as the particles in space and time that are the building blocks of atoms and molecules."

9. David Falk, "New Support for Alternative Quantum View," *Quanta Magazine*, May 16, 2016, quantamagazine.org/pilot-wave-theory-gains-experimental-support-20160516/.

10. Candace Pert, *Molecules of Emotion: The Science Behind Mind-Body Medicine* (New York: Simon & Schuster, 1997).

11. Isabel Pastor Guzman, "How the Body Keeps the Score: An Interview with Dr. Bessel van der Kolk," *Brain World Magazine*, November 27, 2018, brainworldmagazine.com/how-the-body-keeps-the-score-an-interview-with-dr-bessel-van-der-kolk/.

12. Renee Linklater, *Decolonizing Trauma Work: Indigenous Stories and Strategies* (Halifax, Nova Scotia: Fernwood Publishing, 2014). "Indigenous people have lived in a multi-trauma context, meaning that the trauma is personal, collective and historical."

13. Pete Walker, *Complex PTSD: From Surviving to Thriving* (Contra Costa, CA: California Azure Coyote, 2013).

14. "Adverse Childhood Experiences," Substance Abuse and Mental Health Services Administration, July 9, 2018, samhsa.gov/capt/practicing-effective-prevention/prevention-behavioral-health/adverse-childhood-experiences.

15. Sebastian Montes, "Facing a Rising Tide of Personality Disorders," *Counseling Today*, Nov. 1, 2013, ct.counseling.org/2013/11/facing-a-rising-tide-of-personality-disorders/.

16. Nora Weeks, *The Medical Discoveries of Edward Bach Physician* (Oxfordshire, ENG: The C.W. Daniel Company Limited, 1940), 17, 21.

17. Weeks, *The Medical Discoveries of Edward Bach Physician*, 17, 21.

18. "Mental Health Advocacy Fact Sheet," World Health Organization, who.int/mental_health/advocacy/en/#Factsheets.

19. Sara G. Miller, "1 in 6 Americans Takes a Psychiatric Drug," *Scientific American*, December 13, 2016, scientificamerican.com/article/1-in-6-americans-takes-a-psychiatric-drug/.

20. Pema Chödrön, *When Things Fall Apart: Heart Advice for Difficult Times* (Boulder, CO: Shambhala, 2000).

21. Rachel Yehuda, "How Trauma and Resilience Cross Generations," *On Being*, July 30, 2015, onbeing.org/programs/rachel-yehuda-how-trauma-and-resilience-cross-generations/.

22. Jane Bell, in interview with author about Focusing, April 12, 2014.

23. Ann Weiser Cornell, *The Power of Focusing* (New York: MFJ Books, 1996).

24. Alan Watts, *The Wisdom of Insecurity: A Message for an Age of Anxiety* (New York: Random House, 2011).

25. Tom Kenyon, from a lecture on spatial cognizance, October 2017, Seattle, WA.

26. Shawna Wakefield and Teresa Pasquale Mateus, "Conversations in Healing Justice," November 8, 2017, in *Healing Justice Podcast* hosted by Kate Werning, healingjustice.podbean.com/e/ep-2-shawna-teresa-conversation/.

27. Juliet Haines, Sacred Sexual Workshop, 2018, New York, NY.

28. Loretta Pyles, *Healing Justice: Holistic Self-Care for Change Makers* (New York: Oxford University Press, 2018).

29. Pyles, *Healing Justice*.

30. Jack Kornfield, from a lecture from Open Your Heart in Paradise retreat, 2018, Maui, HI.

CHAPTER 3: THE BLOOMS

1. "Traditional, Complementary and Integrative Medicine," World Health Organization, accessed July 20, 2019, who.int/traditional-complementary-integrative-medicine/about/en/.

2. "Complementary, Alternative, or Integrative Health: What's in a Name?" National Center for Complementary and Integrative Health, accessed July 20, 2019, nccih.nih.gov/health/integrative-health.

3. "Complementary, Alternative, or Integrative Health."

4. Gurudas, *Flower Essences and Vibrational Healing*, 2nd ed. (Cassandra Press, 1986).

5. "Perelandra Essences," Perelandra Center for Nature Research, accessed July 22, 2019, perelandra-ltd.com/Perelandra-Essences-C809.aspx.

6. "FAQ," Findhorn Flower Essences, accessed July 22, 2019, findhornessences.com/faq/.

7. "An Interview with Bram Zaalberg, Creator of the Bloesem Remedies Nederland (Flower Essences of the Netherlands), at the International Flower Essence Conferences in Brazil, 2004," Luminesce, accessed July 22, 2019, luminesce.ca/Interview-Flower-Essences-The-Netherlands.html.

8. Claudia Keel, lecture on flowers essences, Arbor Vitae School of Traditional Herbalism, October, 2014, New York, NY.

9. Julian Barnard. *Bach Flower Remedies: Form and Function* (Great Barrington, MA: Lindisfarne, 2002).

10. Patricia Kaminski, *Flowers That Heal: How to Use Flower Essences* (London: New Leaf, 1998).

11. Shantree Kacera, "Herbal Energtics in Clinical Practice: An Energetic Model in Applying the Healing Tastes for Western Herbalism," The Living Centre, accessed July 22, 2019, thelivingcentre.com/herbalism-articles/herbal-energetics-in-clinical-practice-an-energetic-model-in-applying-the-healing-tastes-for-western-herbalism.

12. Karyn Sanders, "Native American Energetics of Healing," lecture, Arbor Vitae School of Traditional Herbalism, January 28 and 29, 2017, New York, NY.

13. Jeffrey Sommer, "The Shanidar IV 'Flower Burial': A Re-evaluation of Neanderthal Burial Ritual," *Cambridge Archaeological Journal* 9, no. 1 (1999): 127–129.

14. John N. Walton et al., *The Oxford Medical Companion* (Oxford: Oxford University Press, 1994).

15. Paul U. Unschuld, *Medicine in China: A History of Ideas* (Berkeley: University of California Press, 1985).

16. Patricia Kaminski and Richard Katz, *Flower Essence Repertory: A Comprehensive Guide to North American and English Flower Essences for Emotional and Spiritual Well-Being* (Nevada City, CA: Flower Essence Society, 1994).

17. Stephen Harrod Buhner, *The Secret Teachings of Plants: The Intelligence of the Heart in the Direct Perception of Nature* (Rochester, VT: Bear & Company, 2004).

18. Jim English, "The Positive Health Benefits of Negative Ions," Nutrition Review, April 22, 2013, nutritionreview.org/2013/04/positive-health-benefits-negative-ions.

19. R. Mandelbaum, lecture on effects of forest bathing on the central nervous system, ArborVitae School of Traditional Herbalism, September 2016, New York, NY.

20. James L. Oschman, *Energy Medicine: The Scientific Basis,* 1st ed. (Edinburgh: Churchill Livingstone, 2000).

21. Richard Gerber, *Vibrational Medicine: The #1 Handbook of Subtle Energy Therapies* (Rochester, VT: Bear & Company, 2001).

22. Steve Johnson, *The Essence of Healing: A Guide to the Alaskan Essences*, 2nd ed. (Homer, AK: Alaskan Flower Essence Project, 2000).

23. Ilya Prigogine and Isabelle Stengers, *Order Out of Chaos: Man's New Dialogue with Nature* (Brooklyn: Verso Books, 2018).

24. Malcolm Gladwell, *The Tipping Point: How Little Things Can Make a Big Difference* (Boston: Little, Brown, 2000).

25. Oschman, *Energy Medicine.*

26. Lata Chettri-Kennedy, email conversation with author, March 1, 2019.

27. Sharla M .Fett, *Working Cures: Healing Health and Power on Southern Slave Plantations* (Chapel Hill: University of North Carolina Press, 2002), 45–52.

28. Barbara Ehrenreich and Deirdre English, *Witches, Midwives, and Nurses: A History of Women Healers*, 2nd ed. (New York: The Feminist Press at CUNY, 1970).

29. "Liz Migliorelli (Sister Spinster) on Decolonizing Your Roots, Holy Waters, Sex Magic & Flower Spells," February 16, 2017, on Dream Freedom Beauty (podcast), 1:21:40, dreamfreedombeauty.com/liz-migliorelli-sister_spinster-on-decolonizing-your-roots-holy-waters-sex-magic-flower-spells-episode-53/?.

30. Julia Graves, *The Language of Plants: A Guide to the Doctrine of Signatures* (Great Barrington, MA: Lindisfarne Books, 2012).

31. Barnard, *Bach Flower Remedies.*

32. Kaminski, *Flowers that Heal*; Graves, *The Language of Plants.*

33. David Dalton, *Delta Gardens Repertory* (catalog) (Hampton Falls, NH: Delta Gardens, October 2016).

34. Philippe Andrianne, *Treatise on Gemmotherapy: The Therapeutic Use of Buds* (Brussels: Editions Amyris, 2012).

35. Graves, *The Language of Plants*.

36. David Dalton, Workshop on Introduction to Flower Essences, May 17, 2014, New York, NY.

37. Kaminski, *Flowers That Heal*.

38. M. Paradise, *Witches, Pagans, and Cultural Appropriation: Considerations and Applications for Magical Practice* (The Anchor & The Star, 2016).

39. Friedwart Husemann, "Bach Flower Remedies in Relation to Anthroposophic Medicine," AnthroMed Library, 1994, anthromed.org/Article.aspx?artpk=256.

40. Deborah Craydon and Warren Bellows, *Floral Acupuncture: Applying the Flower Essences of Dr. Bach to Acupuncture Sites* (Berkeley, CA: Crossing Press, 2005).

41. Sara Crow, "Dew and Flower Essences," Floracopeia, accessed July 22, 2019, floracopeia.com/dew-and-flower-essences.

42. Lawrence Newcomb, *Newcomb's Wildflower Guide: An Ingenious New Key System for Quick, Positive Field Identification of the Wildflowers, Flowering Shrubs and Vines of Northeastern and North-Central North America* (Boston: Little, Brown, 1989); Steven Foster and James A. Duke, *A Field Guide to Medicinal Plants and Herbs of Eastern and Central North American*, 3rd ed. (Boston: Houghton Mifflin Co., 2014).

43. "The Cultural Unity of Black Africa," *Queering Herbalism Encyclopedia, Volume III, Women, Feminine Healing Energy, and Resistance—NYC Feminist Zine Fest Special Edition, Part I* (PDF), etsy.com/listing/215705590/queering-herbalism-encyclopedia-volume-3.

44. Joshua J. Mark, "Female Physicians in Ancient Egypt," Ancient History Encyclopedia, February 22, 2017, ancient.eu/article/49/.

45. Mark, "Female Physicians in Ancient Egypt."

46. Max Dashú, "Woman Shaman," Suppressed Histories Archive, accessed July 22, 2019, suppressedhistories.net/articles/womanshaman.html.

47. Keith Dowman, *Sky Dancer: The Secret Life and Songs of the Lady Yeshe Tsogyel* (Ithaca, NY: Snow Lion, 1996).

48. W. L. Minkowski, "Women Healers of the Middle Ages: Selected Aspects of Their History," *American Journal of Public Health* 82, no. 2 (February 1992): 288–295.

49. Elisabeth Brooke, *Women Healers: Portraits of Herbalists, Physicians, and Midwives* (Rochester, VT: Healing Arts Press, 1995).

50. Ehrenreich and English, *Witches, Midwives, and Nurses.*

51. Alex Owen, *The Darkened Room: Women, Power and Spiritualism in Late Victorian England* (Chicago: University of Chicago Press, 1989).

52. Lorena Hernandez and Vanessa Garcia, "Mujeres, Healing and Autonomy: Reclaiming Our Bodies Means Restoring Indigenous Wellness Practices and Healing Ceremonies," Environmental and Food Justice (blog), March 15, 2013, ejfood.blogspot.com/2013/03/autonomy-body-and-resurgence-of.html.

53. Mama Sarahn Henderson, "The Cauling of Midwife: A Historical Journey of Midwifery Through the Hands of Midwives of African Descent," *Queering Herbalism Encyclopedia, Volume III, Women, Feminine Healing Energy and Resistance—NYC Feminist Zine Fest Special Edition, Part I* (PDF), etsy.com/listing/215705590/queering-herbalism-encyclopedia-volume-3.

54. "Night Vision," Caring Voice Coalition, December 10, 2013, caringvoice.org/2013/12/night-vision/ via Toi Scott vol III.

55. Matthew Wood, *Vitalism: The History of Herbalism, Homeopathy, and Flower Essences* (Berkeley, CA: North Atlantic Books, 2000).

56. Manly P. Hall, *Paracelsus, His Mystical and Medical Philosophy* (Los Angeles: Philosophical Research Society, 1990).

57. Anna M. Stoddart, *The Life of Paracelsus* (London: J. Murray, 1911), 12, 74.

58. Ehrenreich and English, *Witches, Midwives, and Nurses.*

59. Wood, *Vitalism*, 15.

60. Rudolf Steiner, *The Reappearance of Christ in the Etheric* (New York: Steiner Books, 1983).

61. Ray McDermott, "Racism and Waldorf Education," The Online Waldorf Library, accessed July 22, 2019, waldorflibrary.org/images/stories/Journal_Articles/RB1201.pdf.

62. Edward Bach, *Ye Suffer From Yourselves* (Oxon UK: The Bach Centre, 2015), bachcentre.com/centre/download/index.htm.

63. Edward Bach, *Heal Thyself* (Pilgrims Publishing, 2004).

64. Bach, *Heal Thyself*.

65. Peter Damian, *The Twelve Healers of the Zodiac: The Astrology Handbook of the Bach Flower Therapies* (York Beach, ME: S. Weiser, 1986).

66. Bach, *Heal Thyself*.

67. Matthew T. Kapstein, *The Presence of Light: Divine Radiance and Religious Experience* (Chicago: University of Chicago Press, 2004).

68. Doreen Virtue, "Is Your Kid a Rainbow Child?" You Can Heal Your Life, August 24, 2010, healyourlife.com/is-your-kid-a-rainbow-child.

69. David Seamon and Arthur Zajonc, *Goethe's Way of Science: A Phenomenology of Nature* (Albany: State University of New York Press, 1998).

70. Johann Wolfgang von Goethe, *Theory of Colors* (Cambridge, MA: MIT Press, 1970).

71. Workshop on Color Theory and Flower Essences, Flower Essence Society, August 2016, Nevada City, CA.

72. Anne McIntyre, *Flower Power: Flower Remedies for Healing Body and Soul Through Herbalism, Homeopathy, Aromatherapy, and Flower Essences* (New York: Henry Holt, 1996).

73. Loren Eiseley, *How Flowers Changed the World* (New York: Random House, 1996).

74. Carlo Rovelli, *Reality Is Not What It Seems: The Journey to Quantum Reality* (New York: Riverhead Books 2017), 60.

CHAPTER 4: FLOWER RITUALS FOR HEALING AND TRANSFORMATION

1. Julian Barnard, *Bach Flower Remedies: Form and Function* (Great Barrington, MA: Lindisfarne, 2002).

2. Loren Eiseley, *How Flowers Changed the World* (New York: Random House, 1996).

3. Eugen Strouhal, *Life of the Ancient Egyptians* (Norman: University of Oklahoma Press, 1992).

4. Keith Critchlow, *The Hidden Geometry of Flowers: Living Rhythms, Form and Number* (Edinburgh: Floris Books, 2011).

5. Anne McIntyre, *Flower Power: Flower Remedies for Healing Body and Soul Through Herbalism, Homeopathy, Aromatherapy, and Flower Essences* (New York: Henry Holt, 1996).

6. Brian Froud and Alan Lee, *Faeries* (New York: Harry N. Abrams, 1978).

7. Philippe Andrienne, *Treatise on Gemmotherapy: The Therapeutic Use of Buds* (Brussels: Editions Amyris, 2012).

8. Rosita Arvigo and Nadine Epstein, *Spiritual Bathing: Healing Rituals and Traditions from Around the World* (Battleboro, VT: Echo Point Books & Media, 2018).

9. Julia Graves, *The Language of Plants: A Guide to the Doctrine of Signatures* (Great Barrington, MA: Lindisfarne Books, 2012).

10. Loretta Pyles, *Healing Justice: Holistic Self-Care for Change Makers* (Oxford: Oxford University Press, 2018).

11. James L. Oschman et al., "The Effects of Grounding (Earthing) on Inflammation, the Immune Response, Wound Healing, and Prevention and Treatment of Chronic Inflammatory and Autoimmune Diseases," *Journal of Inflammation Research* 8 (2015): 83–96, doi:10.2147/JIR.S69656.

12. Robert Simmons, Naisha Ahsian, and Hazel Raven, *The Book of Stones: Who They Are and What They Teach* (Berkeley, CA: North Atlantic Books, 2007).

13. Anne Harrington, *Mind Fixers: Psychiatry's Troubled Search for the Biology of Mental Illness* (Grand Haven, MI: Brilliance Audio, 2019).

14. Mechthild Scheffer, *Encyclopedia of Bach Flower Therapy* (Rochester, VT: Healing Arts Press, 2001).

15. Scheffer, *Encyclopedia of Bach Flower Therapy*.

16. Mary O'Malley, *What's in the Way Is the Way: A Practical Guide for Waking Up to Life* (Boulder, CO: Sounds True, 2016).

17. *Diagnostic and Statistical Manual of Mental Disorders*, 5th ed. (Arlington, VA: American Psychiatric Publishing, 2013).

18. Renee Linklater, *Decolonizing Trauma Work: Indigenous Stories and Strategies* (Halifax, Nova Scotia: Fernwood Publishing, 2014).

19. Modern Women, *Many Moons 2018 Vol 2: July–December* (Los Angeles: Many Moons Publications, 2018).

20. "2015 Heart Disease and Stroke Statistics Update," American Heart Association, December 17, 2014, heart.org/idc/groups/ahamah-public/@wcm/@sop/@smd/documents/downloadable/ucm_470704.pdf. "Cardiovascular disease is the leading global cause of death, accounting for 17.3 million deaths per year."

21. Frank Wilczek, "Entanglement Made Simple," *Quanta Magazine*, April 28, 2016, quantamagazine.org/entanglement-made-simple-20160428/; Jon Cartwright, "Collapse: Has Quantum Theory's Greatest Mystery Been Solved?" *New Scientist*, July 16, 2016, landing.newscientist.com/department-for-education-feature-3/.

22. "Scientific Foundation of the HeartMath System," HeartMath Institute, accessed February 22, 2019, heartmath.org/science/.

23. T. L. Goldsby, M. E. Goldsby, M. McWalters, et al., "Effects of Singing Bowl Sound Meditation on Mood, Tension, and Well-Being: An Observational Study," *Journal of Evidence-Based Complementary & Alternative Medicine* 22, no. 3 (2017): 401–406, doi:10.1177/2156587216668109.

24. "Pets: Making a Connection That's Healthy for Humans," HeartMath Institute, April 23, 2010, heartmath.org/articles-of-the-heart/social-connections/pets-making-a-connection-thats-healthy-for-humans/.

25. *APA Monitor* 31, no. 7, 2000.

26. Shelley E. Taylor et al., "Biobehavioral Responses to Stress in Females: Tend-and-Befriend, Not Fight-or-Flight," *Psychological Review* 107, no. 3 (2000), 411–429.

Glossary

Alchemy: An inner process of transformation.

Alignment: The process of coming into cosmic balance, a state of harmony within the self and in one's environment, also known as *ascending*.

Anthroposophy: Complementary healing approach blending traditional and alternative methods to support mind-body-spirit balance and health; founded by Rudolf Steiner in the 1920s.

Ascension: Process of soul evolution and coming into *alignment*; occurs across multiple lifetimes and happens in tandem with the collective and all life.

Astral body: Composed of *astral matter*, this is a subtle substance of even higher energetic frequencies than etheric matter. The emotional body is part of the *chakra system*. It governs desires and fears and is connected to the physical body via the *etheric body*. It can be engaged when a person is asleep, and it is associated with near-death experiences, out-of-body experiences, and astral projection.

Astral subtle matter: Highly magnetic, attracting and repelling energy.

Attachment style: Type of care we receive from our caregivers as infants and children; corresponds to how we feel in relationship with ourselves, with others, and our world. There are four types of attachment: secure, anxious, avoidant, and disorganized.

Attunement: The process of making deep contact with another realm or spirit, usually a plant or stone; e.g., attuning with a plant allows one to connect with the consciousness of that plant spirit, gaining insight into how it works, how it wants to help, etc.

Bypass: The process of sub- or unconsciously avoiding dealing with an issue, usually because tolerating the distress is too painful.

Capitalism: A patriarchal economic system wherein a group's trade and industry are privately owned, instead of publicly owned; a system of scarcity that rewards the dominant culture.

Causal body (also *spiritual body*): Exists in the frequency range beyond the *mental body*; stores all lifetime experiences acquired in the reincarnation system.

Chakra system: A system of energy centers along the central axis of the body that are connected to both the *physical* and *subtle bodies* via energetic pathways; they are also connected with the meridians and nadis. There are perhaps seven chakras: root, sacral, solar plexus, heart, throat, third eye, and crown. This system closely resembles the hormonal centers of the endocrine system.

Co-creation: Conscious, intentional creation in the flow with life, as opposed to *egoic* or *unconscious creation*.

Collective consciousness: The shared beliefs and psycho-spiritual functioning level of the general population.

Consciousness: A state of awareness that can occur in multiple levels and dimensions simultaneously and is not limited by time or space. Everything with a vibrational signature possesses consciousness—this includes but is not limited to the elements, the ocean, the cosmos, places, memories, disease, feeling states, plants, stones, and animals.

Cosmic: Relating to the Universe and the governing principles held therein.

Crystalline network: Biocrystalline structures that form a network within the body and are made up of interstitial fluid, cell salts, fatty tissues, lymph tissue, red and white blood cells, and the pineal gland. These physical structures interact with the *subtle bodies* to orchestrate the distribution of vibrational medicines.

Cultural appropriation: The stealing or borrowing from a culture—usually by a member of a dominant culture from a minority culture—without asking for permission, giving credit, or offering compensation; something taken inappropriately for one's own personal gain, and can include artwork, intellectual property, and practices.

Decolonization: The act of restoring a group or practice's independence and sovereignty.

Deva: The archetypal spiritual intelligence behind a species; can also apply to an individual, place, or situation.

Discernment: The practice of synchronizing the heart, mind, and higher knowing to make decisions and energetic investments.

Dismantling: The act of taking apart harmful structures, such as belief systems.

Divine feminine consciousness: The sacred characteristics of the feminine; the feminine in its exalted state, transcending egoic identification; also associated with fourth, and more often fifth, dimensional consciousness.

Divine masculine consciousness: The sacred characteristics of the masculine; the masculine in its exalted state, transcending egoic identification; also associated with fourth, and more often fifth, dimensional consciousness.

Duality: Binary of opposites; dual thinking holds that something must be either/or, instead of and; e.g., something can be shadow *or* light.

Egoic feminine consciousness: The current general collective consciousness associated with the feminine; identified at the level of ego, also with the third dimension.

Egoic masculine consciousness: The current general collective consciousness associated with the masculine; identified at the level of ego, also with the third dimension.

Elements: Arising out of the ancient Greek and Asian concepts for air, earth, fire, and water; each has a corresponding spirit, called an "elemental."

Empath: A highly sensitive individual who may have enhanced clairvoyant, clairaudient, and/or clairsentient abilities; individuals especially vulnerable to taking on the negative effect, conflict, and/or suffering of other beings and the collective.

Energetic: The energy or vibrational nature surrounding or underlying something.

Energetic dose: An extremely low dose of 1–5 drops, usually of an herbal tincture, also sometimes referred to as a spirit dose.

Energetics: Relating to a plant's therapeutic actions; i.e., relaxing, stimulating, dispersing, etc.

Etheric body: Forms the blueprint for the *physical body*'s health and/or illness. In death, the etheric body separates from the person and returns as free energy to the Universe.

Etheric matter: Referred to in Eastern esoteric literature as subtle matter; less dense, or of a higher frequency, than physical matter.

Etheric subtle energy: Energy that exists at a higher octave level (*frequency*) than the physical body.

Fifth dimension: The domain of consciousness we will ascend into that exists beyond the level of ego. Some characteristics of this dimension include unconditional love, instant manifestation, cosmic balance, and unity consciousness.

Flower essence: A vibrational plant medicine made from flowers placed in water and a small amount of preservative, such as brandy. Flower essences do not contain physical plant constituents as do herbal tinctures or teas, but they contain the energetic blueprint or vibratory signature of the plant. They can be used to address a wide variety of emotional, mental, and spiritual, as well as physical conditions and situations.

Flower of life: Sacred symbol depicting nineteen overlapping circles; some feel it represents Source and the creation of all life; it contains numerous sacred geometric codes including the tree of life and Metatron's cube.

Fourth dimension: The domain of consciousness many of us are currently ascending into; the awareness of both ego and soul. Some characteristics of this dimension include presence, seeing the relationship between thought and reality, nonduality, and expanded consciousness.

Frequency: A vibrational measurement. Rule of thumb: the higher the frequency of matter, the less dense or more subtle the matter. Divided into octaves, all matter has frequency. Matter of different frequencies can coexist in the same space.

Grounding: A protective and restorative practice that is the process of attuning one's energy with the Earth's frequency; can be enhanced by utilizing breath work, visualization, and flower essences.

Healing justice: A concept introduced by Cara Page of the Kindred Southern Healing Justice Collective that "identifies how we can holistically respond to and intervene on generational trauma and violence, and to bring collective practices that can impact and transform the consequences of oppression on our bodies, hearts and minds" (incite-national.org/2010/08/05/reflections-from-detroit-transforming-wellness-wholeness/). It is informed by a long history of political liberatory frameworks—racial justice, economic justice, reproductive justice, disability justice, and transformative justice, among others—that recognize how systemic oppression, violence, and trauma impact us on both an individual and collective level and also the role of resilience in healing.

Holographic principle: A theoretical framework that holds that every piece contains the whole and can create an energy interference pattern; every cell within the human body contains the information to create an entire duplicate body; "As above, so below."

Intention: The declaration, goal, or vision for a desired outcome.

Intersectionality: The interconnectedness of gender, sexual orientation, race, class, ability, and culture.

Institutional racism: Racism expressed systemically at the sociopolitical level that informs the disparity around health care, income, and criminal justice, among other factors; can be difficult to observe due to its ingrained and subtle characteristics within the dominant culture.

Light body: The sacred geometrical light framework around the Self that connects the *physical body* and *subtle bodies* with the cosmos.

Light worker: One who intentionally engages light in their healing practice; one who is intentionally working to bring light into the planet; one who seeks to evolve beyond the level of ego and be of service.

Lunaception: The process of synchronizing one's menstrual cycle with the moon.

Macrocosm: The whole system; also Universe or cosmos; the macrocosm has a reciprocal relationship with the microcosm.

Manifestation: The process of encouraging a desired outcome through intention.

Matriarchy: A system ruled by and organized around women.

Mental body: Exists in the frequency range beyond the *astral body*; comprises thought forms, ideas, sensations, and beliefs.

Microcosm: Part of the whole; humans are a part of the Universe; the microcosm has a reciprocal relationship with the *macrocosm*.

Misogyny: Ingrained hatred and prejudices against women and the feminine; the world's current dominant systems function in large part as a result of systemic misogyny.

Mystery schools: An ancient collective, or school, with its own sacred teachings; the wisdom of these schools is handed down through various lineages for the purpose of evolution and ascension.

Nonduality (or nondualism): Terms that originate from Buddhist, Hindu, Taoist, many indigenous and shamanic teachings, and various esoteric and mystical texts; means oneness.

Patriarchy: A system ruled by and organized around men; the current pervading system of power in our world.

Physical body: The gross, corporeal self; depends on the *etheric body* for survival.

Plant signature: The way in which a plant has adapted to its environment and assumes certain forms; the plant's personality.

Polarity: One of two sides of something; can be positive or negative.

Program: A set of internalized beliefs we interpret as true; determines much of how we function.

Quantum healing: Changes in consciousness result in profound healing of the mind, body, and spirit, as introduced by Deepak Chopra in his book, *Quantum Healing*.

Quantum mechanics: Also sometimes referred to as quantum physics, a scientific framework which aims to define physical phenomena beyond the subatomic level.

Rainbow body: Within the Tibetan Buddhist tradition, an ultimate state of enlightenment wherein a person's soul turns rainbow and then becomes pure light.

Ritual: An intentional practice with a therapeutic purpose.

Sacred geometry: Refers to the patterns found within structures of the natural world as well as in human-made structures of sacred art and architecture; correlates to the harmonics, or resonant frequencies, found in music, light, and cosmology.

Shadow work: Engaging part of the unconscious, or shadow, for greater integration and healing.

Starseed: An individual who feels they have incarnated into Earth from a star realm or other part of the Universe; associated with Indigo, Rainbow, and Crystal children and individuals; usually shares many characteristics with empaths.

Subconscious: Between the conscious and the unconscious; what has been suppressed.

Subtle: Referring to energy, matter, and the bodies at a higher frequency or resonance than the physical, more dense level.

Subtle body/bodies: Those psycho-spiritual planes of the self that exist outside the physical body, including the etheric, astral, mental, and causal; they are distinct layers but are connected via energetic pathways.

Third dimension: Current general level of collective consciousness; identified at the level of ego; characteristics of this dimension include survival consciousness, duality, and density.

Thought forms: Conscious or unconscious thoughts existing in the astral and mental body; may have emotional intensity, making them denser.

Tissue state: In herbalism, the term which defines how physical structures function; the six tissue states are hot, cold, dry, damp, constriction, and relaxation.

Transpersonal psychology: Branch of psychology developed by Carl Jung that explores healing and reality outside the self, or physical body, and integrates the spiritual aspects of the self and the human experience.

Unconscious: What we don't know; deep in the void.

Vibrational: The energetic quality of something; associated with and can be measured at the level of frequency; term is sometimes used interchangeably with *energetic* and *subtle energetic*.

Vibrational medicine: Sometimes called subtle energetic medicine; uses specialized forms of energy to positively affect those energetic systems that may be out of balance due to disease states.

Vitalism: Energy that inhabits and influences the physical body; similar to the concept of qi in traditional Chinese medicine, prana in Ayurveda, and vital force in homeopathy, *ashé* in Yoruba.

White privilege: In Western societies, the sociopolitical and economic benefits white people enjoy that are unearned; these benefits are generally hidden and unconsciously inherent to the values and beliefs of the dominant culture.

Resources

ANCIENT EGYPT

El Zeini, Hanny and Catherine Dees. *Omm Sety's Egypt: A Story of Ancient Mysteries, Secret Lives, and the Lost History of the Pharaohs.* Pittsburgh, PA: St. Lynn's Press, 2007.

Ellis, Normandi. *Awakening Osiris: The Egyptian Book of the Dead.* Cork: Red Wheel Weiser, 2009.

———*Dreams of Isis: A Woman's Spiritual Sojourn.* Wheaton, IL: Quest Books, 1995.

Tyldesley, Joyce A. *Daughters of Isis: Women of Ancient Egypt.* London: Penguin Books, 1995.

West, John Anthony. *Serpent in the Sky: The High Wisdom of Ancient Egypt.* London: Wilwood House, 1979.

———*The Traveler's Key to Ancient Egypt: A Guide to the Sacred Places of Ancient Egypt.* Wheaton, IL: Quest Books, 1995.

FEMININE CONSCIOUSNESS AND THE LUNAR REALM

Adler, Margot. *Drawing Down the Moon: Witches, Druids, Goddess-Worshippers, and Other Pagans in America.* New York: Penguin Books, 2014.

Canty, Jeanine M., ed. *Ecological and Social Healing: Multicultural Women's Voices.* New York: Routledge, 2017.

Cashford, Jules. *The Moon: Myth and Image.* London: Cassell Illustrated, 2003.

de Beauvoir, Simone. *The Second Sex.* London: Vintage Classic, 2015.

Ehrenreich, Barbara and Deirdre English. *Witches, Midwives, and Nurses: A History of Women Healers.* New York: The Feminist Press at CUNY, 2010.

Estés, Clarissa Pinkola. *Women Who Run with the Wolves: Myths and Stories of the Wild Woman Archetype.* New York: Ballantine Books, 2003.

Federici, Silvia. *Caliban and the Witch: Woman, the Body and Primitive Accumulation.* New York: Autonomedia, 2004.

Friedan, Betty. *The Feminine Mystique*. New York: W. W. Norton, 2013.

Holland, Jack. *Misogyny: The Oldest Prejudice in the World*. Philadelphia: Running Press, 2007.

Hooks, Bell. *Ain't I a Woman?: Black Women and Feminism*. New York: Routledge, 2014.

McKenzie, Mia. *Black Girl Dangerous: On Race, Queerness, Class, and Gender*. Oakland: BGD Press, Inc., 2014.

Rush, Anne Kent. *Moon, Moon*. Daphe, AL: Moon Books, 2014.

Steinem, Gloria. *Revolution from Within: A Book of Self-Esteem*. New York: Corgi, 2012.

Wolf, Naomi. *Vagina: A New Biography*. London: Virago, 2012.

VIBRATIONAL HEALING

Emoto, Masaru, translated by David A. Thayne. *The Hidden Messages in Water*. New York: Atria Books, 2005.

Gerber, Richard. *Vibrational Medicine: The #1 Handbook of Subtle-Energy Therapies*. Rochester, VT: Bear & Company, 2001.

Gurudas. *Flower Essences and Vibrational Healing*. Albuquerque, NM: Brotherhood of Life, 1983.

Kenyon, Tom and Virginia Essene. *The Hathor Material: Messages from an Ascended Civilization*. Santa Clara, CA: S.E.E. Pub. Co., 1996.

Oschman, James L. *Energy Medicine: The Scientific Basis*. Edinburgh: Elsevier, 2016.

Talbot, Michael and Lynne McTaggart. *The Holographic Universe: The Revolutionary Theory of Reality*. New York: Harper Perennial, 2011.

FLOWER ESSENCES

Barnard, Julian. *Bach Flower Remedies: Form and Function*. Great Barrington, MA: Lindisfarne, 2002.

Barnard, Julian., ed. *Collected Writings of Edward Bach: The Man Who Discovered the Bath Flower Remedies*. Bath: Ashgrove Press, 1998.

Dalton, David. *Stars of the Meadow: Medicinal Herbs as Flower Essences.* Great Barrington, MA: Lindisfarne Books, 2013.

Graves, Julia. *The Language of Plants: A Guide to the Doctrine of Signatures.* Great Barrington, MA: Lindisfarne Books, 2012.

Gurudas. *Flower Essences and Vibrational Healing.* Albuquerque, NM: Brotherhood of Life, 1983.

Johnson, Steve. *The Essence of Healing: A Guide to the Alaskan Essences.* Homer, AK: Alaskan Flower Essence Project, 2000.

Kaminski, Patricia. *Flowers That Heal: How to Use Flower Essences.* London: New Leaf, 1998.

Kaminski, Patricia and Richard Katz. *Flower Essence Repertory: A Comprehensive Guide to North American and English Flower Essences for Emotional and Spiritual Well-Being.* Nevada City, CA: Flower Essence Society, 1994.

McIntyre, Anne. *Flower Power: Flower Remedies for Healing Body and Soul Through Herbalism, Homeopathy, Aromatherapy, and Flower Essences.* New York: Henry Holt and Co., 1996.

Scheffer, Mechthild. *Bach Flower Therapy: Theory and Practice.* London: Thorsons, 1990.

———*The Encyclopedia of Bach Flower Therapy.* Rochester, VT: Healing Arts Press, 2001.

Small Wright, Machaelle. *Flower Essences: Reordering our Understanding and Our Approach to Illness and Health.* Jeffersonton, VA: Perelandra, 1988.

Weeks, Nora and Victor Bullen. *The Bach Flower Remedies: Illustration and Preparation.* London: Ebury Digital, 2012.

Wood, Matthew. *Vitalism: The History of Herbalism, Homeopathy, and Flower Essences.* Berkeley, CA: North Atlantic Books, 2000.

CLINICAL FLOWER ESSENCE RESEARCH

Bach Educational Resource, bacheducationalresource.org/en/.

Flower Essence Society, flowersociety.org/ejournals-links.htm.

HEALING AND SOCIAL JUSTICE

AORTA—Anti-Oppression Resource and Training Alliance, aorta.coop.

The Audre Lorde Project, alp.org.

Bad Ass Visionary Healers, badassvisionaryhealers.wordpress.com/healing-justice-principles/.

Black Lives Matter, blacklivesmatter.com.

Bron, Taylor. "Earthen Spirituality or Cultural Genocide? Radical Environmentalism's Appropriation of Native American Spirituality." *Religion* 27, no. 2 (April 1997).

Catalyst Project, collectiveliberation.org.

Coates, Ta-Nehisi. "The Case for Reparations." *The Atlantic*, June 2014.

Competent Care for Transgender, GenderQueer, and Non-Binary Folks, sites.google.com/vtherbcenter.org/transhealth/home.

DiAngelo, Robin. *White Fragility: Why It's So Hard for White People to Talk About Racism*. Boston: Beacon Press, 2018.

Dorsey, Danielle. "How One Woman is Reclaiming Herbalism as a Form of Resistance." Wear Your Voice, February 3, 2018, wearyourvoicemag.com/culture/herbalism-as-resistance.

Gilio-Whitaker, Dina. "Unpacking the Invisible Knapsack of Settler Privilege." Beacon Broadside, November 8, 2018, beaconbroadside.com/broadside/2018/11/unpacking-the-invisible-knapsack-of-settler-privilege.html.

Healing Justice Podcast, healingjustice.org.

Johnson, Allan G. *Privilege, Power, and Difference*. New York: McGraw-Hill Education, 2018.

Kindred Southern Healing Justice Collective, healingcollectivetrauma.com/kindred-collective-wellness-within-liberation.html.

Leaving Evidence, leavingevidence.wordpress.com/tag/disability-justice.

Linklater, Renee. *Decolonizing Trauma Work: Indigenous Stories and Strategies.* Halifax, Nova Scotia: Fernwood Publishing, 2014; London: Penguin, 2019.

Pyles, Loretta. *Healing Justice: Holistic Self-Care for Change Makers.* Oxford: Oxford University Press, 2018.

Rosenberg, Virginia. "Converting Hidden Spiritual Racism into Sacred Activism: An Open Letter to Spiritual White Folks." July 10, 2016, virginiarosenberg.com/blog/2016/7/10/converting-hidden-spiritual-racism-into-sacred-activism-an-open-letter-to-spiritual-white-folks.

Scott, Toi. "We are the Sum of Our Ancestors: Decolonizing Herbalism." *Decolonizing Yoga*, June 7, 2013, decolonizingyoga.com/we-are-the-sum-of-our-ancestors-decolonizing-herbalism/.

Southerners on New Ground (SONG). "On the Role of White People in the Movement at This Time." southernersonnewground.org/wp-content/uploads/2015/04/White_People_Role_in_this_Time_April2015_WEB.pdf.

Unsettling America: Decolonization in Theory and Practice, unsettlingamerica.wordpress.com.

FLOWER ESSENCE TEACHINGS AND TRAININGS

Alaskan Essences Inc. Practitioner Training Program, alaskanessences.com/pages/practitioner-certification-program.

Bach Educational Resource, bacheducationalresource.org/en/.

Delta Gardens Flower Essences Practitioner Training, deltagardens.com/pages/practitioner-training.

Desert Alchemy Workshops, desert-alchemy.com/workshops/.

Flower Essence Society Classes, flowersociety.org/classes.htm.

Green Tara Essences, lilycircle.com/ workshops/; facebook.com/LilyCircleandGreenTaraFlowerEssences/.

Healing Herbs Bach Flower Learning Programme, bachflowerlearning.com/en/.

Sister Spinster (regularly offers classes on herbalism that occasionally include flower essences), sisterspinster.net/events-classes/.

Index

Italicized page numbers refer to images.

abundance, 144–46
acceptance, 42–43
addiction, 29
Alaskan essences, 89, 95, 128, 136, 184–85
aloe, 63–64
altars, 127, 160
anxiety, 28
astrology, 113–14
auric fields, 68, 141
Ayurvedic medicine and traditions, 31, 57, 62, 69

Bach, Edward, 27, 56–57, 85, 112–15, 117, 183
Bagg, Deborah, 158, 160
balance, 11, 19–20, 31–32, 34
Barnard, Julian, 56, 85, 183
beauty, 72, 146
beliefs, 34–39
Bell, Jane, 1, 12
Bloesem Remedies, 95, 136, 185
Bodhisattva Guanyin (goddess of compassion), *48*
bodies, types of
    emotional body, 28
    subtle body, 57, 68–69, 70–72, 74–75, 134
    vibrational system bodies, 71, *73*, 74–75
breathing, 41–42, 155–58, 176
Buhner, Stephen, 65
bypassing, 153–54

caduceus, 109
capitalism, 14, 105, 196
case studies
    Choosing Conscious Beliefs, 37–38
    How Nature Heals, 65–67
    Synchronicity in the Healing Process, 60–61
Cashford, Jules, 12
Catholicism, 14
centering ritual, 128
chakra system, *33*, 59, 71, 93, *94*
Chettri-Kennedy, Lata, 77

Chinese medicine/traditional Chinese medicine (TCM), 31, 57, 62, 87, 173
choice, 36
collaboration, 145
colonization and cultural appropriation, 78–82
color theory, 116–19
competition, 145
complementary and alternative medicine (CAM), 6–7, 53
conscious beliefs, 34–39
consciousness, 16, 32
    Focusing, 39
    survival consciousness, 41
crystalline network, 74
cultural appropriation and colonization, 78–82

Dalton, David, 148–49
Day of the Dead/*Día de los Muertos*, 163
death and loss, 163–67
decolonization, 79–80
Delta Gardens, 54, 89, 128, 136, 183–84
depression, 28, 164
dew, 100, *101*, 110
Diop, Cheikh Anta, 105
divine feminine, 3–4, 13, 16–18, 46, 76, 145, 148, 198
dream work, 167–70
duality/nonduality, 4, 6, 20–21, *22–23*
    characteristics of, 21
    healing, 23–26

Earth, xi, 4, 13, 138–39, 180
ego, 30, 32, 34, 47, 59, 70, 114, 150, 153–54, 163, 198
Egyptian traditions and practices, 62, 67–68, 129–30
    author's own experience with, 1, 81–82, 122
    balance, 31
    flower of life, 122
    Ma'at, 12, 19
    moon, 12
    Nana Bùrúkú, 12
    Thoth, 109
elements, 87, 89
emotions, 24–26, 28–29

empaths, 45, 151
energetics, 57–59, 66
energy, 52
Energy Medicine: The Scientific Basis (Oschman), 68
epigenetics, 35
equilibrium, 11
exercises
   intention, 9
   Datura flower essence and breath work, 155–58
   plant attunement, 83–84
   rainbow worksheet, 119
   surrender, 55
   see also rituals

fear, 25–26, 30, 41
felt sense, 39
feminine, 3–4, 11–12, 20, 45–46, 55, 175, 198
   divine feminine, 3–4, 13, 16–18, 46, 76, 145, 148, 198
   moon times, 12–14
   yin and yang, 14, *22*, 31, 89
   see also masculine
feminism, 16–17
Findhorn Essences, 56
floriography, 132
flower burial, 62
Flower Essence Services (FES), 183, 185
flower essences, 2, 5–6, 51–56
   Alaskan essences, 89, 95, 128, 136, 184–85
   application, 97
   awareness, 12
   Bloesem Remedies, 95, 136, 185
   change, agents of, 24
   color, 117
   creation and preparation of, 56–57
   cultural appropriation and colonization, 78–82
   defining, 51–52, 55–56
   Delta Gardens, 54, 89, 128, 136, 183–84
   dream work, essences for, 170
   energetics, 57–59
   evaluating effectiveness of, 62
   Findhorn Essences, 56
   foundations of the practice, 110–15
   formulating, 91–92, 98, *99*, 100, 102–3
   green tara flower essences, 184–85
   grief and loss, essences for, 166–67
   healing justice, essences for, 180
   herbal preparations versus flower essences, 67
   how they work, 56–60
   intention, essences for, 143
   lower vibratory states, essences for, 152–53
   menstruation, essences for, 158–60
   moonlight flower essence, 148–49
   online resources, 185
   poisonous plants, working with, 155
   relaxation, essences for, 137–38
   rose essence and heart breathing, 176–77
   rituals, 96–97, 125–28, 141
   safety and protection, 133–38; essences for, 135–37; rituals, 141
   selecting, 89–90
   self-care, 46
   storing, 103–4
   when to use, 94–95
   woodland essences, 184–85
   working with others, 96
   see also flowers and plants
Flower Essences and Vibrational Healing (Gurudas), 2, 55
flower of life, 121–22, 180–81
flowers and plants
   black cohosh, *147*
   Datura, *147*, 155–56, 162
   elements of, 87, 89
   evening primrose, *147*
   flower of life, 121–22, 180–81
   geometry, 87, *88*
   green bells of Ireland, *147*
   history of use in healing traditions, 129–33
   lady's mantle, *101*
   learning about, 82–90
   lotus, 129–30, 132
   mariposa lily, *25*
   mimulus, 1
   moon garden flowers, 162
   morning glory, *58*
   roses, 176–77
   senses, 84–85
   shapes, 85–87
   tobacco, *147*
   see also flower essences
Flowers that Heal (Kaminski, Patricia and Richard), 85
Focusing, 39

forest bathing, 66
frequency, 74

generosity/being of service, 47–48
geometry of plants, 87, *88*
Gilligan, Carol, 16–17
goddesses of the ancient world, 17
Goethe, Johann Wolfgang, *116*, 117
Graves, Julia, 85, 89, 133, 184
grief, 164–67
Groode, David, 1
grounding, 138–39
Gurudas, 2, 55, 97

Hahnemann, Samuel, 111
Haines, Juliet, 46
healers, historical, 105–9
healing, 7, 23–26, 60–61
healing justice, 6–7, 51, 82, 134, 179–80, 200
healing traditions, use of flowers in, 129–33
heart and heart medicine rituals, 172–77
herbal medicine, 52–54, 62–64
  see also flower essences
Hindu traditions, 19, 34, 62, 132
holographic principle, 75
homeopathy, 53–54, 67, 111, 113

intention, 8–9, 60, 91, 142–43

Jung, Carl, 32, 150
justice, 179–80
  see also healing justice

Kali Yuga, 19
Kaminski, Patricia and Richard, 85
Keel, Claudia, 3

The Language of Plants (Graves), 85, 89, 184
Lazarus, Emma, xi
lotus, 129–30, 132
love, 25–26, 42, 174–76

Ma'at, 12, 19
masculine, 11, 55, 145
  programs, 30

sun times, 12–14
yin and yang, 14, *22*, 31, 89
see also feminine
matriarchal societies, 14
Maya, 34
medicine
  complementary and alternative medicine (CAM), 6–7, 53
  herbal medicine, 52–54, 62–64
  Western medicine, 6, 53–54
  see also flower essences; vibrational medicine
menstruation, 158–60
midwifery, 108
moon, 3, 12–14, 76–78, 148–51, 158–60
moon gardens, 160, *161*, 162
The Moon: Myth and Image (Cashford), 12
moon times, 12–14
moonlight flower essence, 148–49
Mourning Dove, 64

Nana Bùrúkú, 12
National Institutes of Health (NIH), 53, 55
Native American traditions and practices, 64, 79, 108, 132–33, 173
nature, healing power of, 64–67
no (saying no), 46
nonduality. See duality/nonduality

oak/*Quercus robur*, 131
Oschman, James L., 68–69

Paracelsus, 81–82, 100, 110–11
Patterson, Jennifer, 155, 158
patriarchy, 11–12, 16, 20, 105, 145
plants. See flowers and plants
presence, 42–43
privilege, 15, 144
programs, 30
PTSD, 27, 164

quantum theory, 19–20, 23, 54, 59, 76, 186–8

rainbows, 116–17, 119, *120*
Ram Dass, 154
relaxation, 43

relaxation, flower essences for, 137–38
rituals, 96–97, 125–28
    bedtime rituals, 169
    grounding, 139
    heart medicine rituals, 172–77
    protective mist, 125–28
    protective rituals, 141
    re-centering, 128
    surrender, 55
    see also exercises
Rumi, 151

safety and protection, 133–38
    essences for, 135–37
    rituals, 141
Salzberg, Sharon, 47
Sanders, Karyn, 57
the self, 32, 150
self-care, 44–46
the senses, 84–85
the shadow and shadow work, 150–58
sleep, 167–70
Steiner, Rudolph, 72, 84, 111–12, 117
storytelling, 30
sun times, 12–14
surrendering, 154–55
synchronicity, 59–61

tend and befriend, 179–80
Thich Nhat Hanh, 49, 150
thought forms, 75
trauma, 7, 27–29
Tubman, Harriet, 109

vibrational medicine, 2, 24–26, 52–54, 67–71
    bodies, 71–72, *73*, 74–75
    frequency, 74
    key terms, 74–75
    lower vibratory states, 24–26, 28–29, 151–53
    the moon, 76–78
    tenets of, 69–70
    see also flower essences

Watson, Lilla, 1
Weeks, Nora, 115
Western medicine, 6, 53–54

white privilege, 15, 144
witches, 107–8
women healers, 105–9
Wright, Machaelle Small, 54, 56

yin and yang, 14, *22*, 31, 89

About the Author

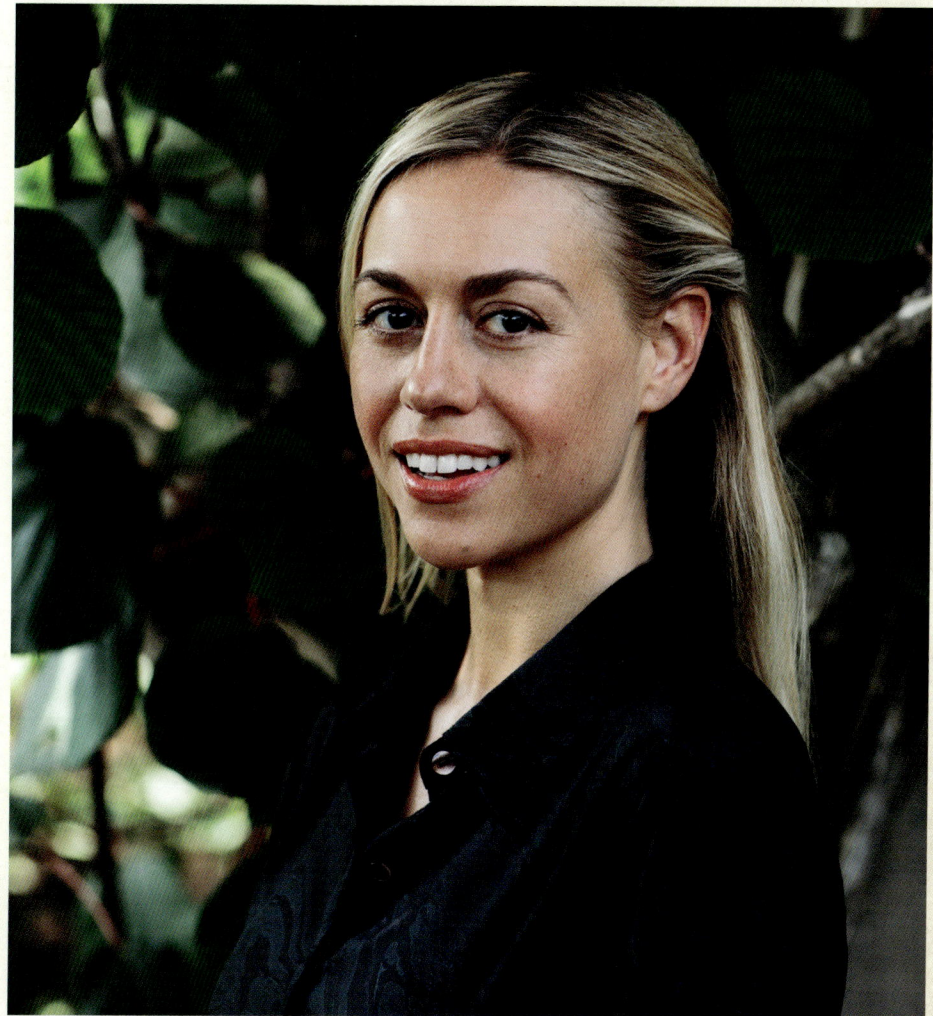

Heidi Smith, MA, RH (AHG), is a therapist, registered herbalist, and flower essence practitioner. Her private practice is called Moon & Bloom, and she is the co-creator of Spirit Shop. She lives in Brooklyn with her partner and two cats.

About Sounds True

Sounds True is a multimedia publisher whose mission is to inspire and support personal transformation and spiritual awakening. Founded in 1985 and located in Boulder, Colorado, we work with many of the leading spiritual teachers, thinkers, healers, and visionary artists of our time. We strive with every title to preserve the essential "living wisdom" of the author or artist. It is our goal to create products that not only provide information to a reader or listener but also embody the quality of a wisdom transmission.

For those seeking genuine transformation, Sounds True is your trusted partner. At SoundsTrue.com you will find a wealth of free resources to support your journey, including exclusive weekly audio interviews, free downloads, interactive learning tools, and other special savings on all our titles.

To learn more, please visit SoundsTrue.com/freegifts or call us toll-free at 800.333.9185.

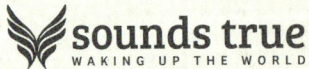